AF589160

‘A notable contribution to understand post-pandemic mental health in India. The qualitative and quantitative mix is robust and caters to both tastes’.

Prof Rajbir Singh, *Adjunct Faculty, Chaudhary Ranbir Singh Institute of Social and Economic Change, MD University, Rohtak, Haryana*

‘The aftermath of pandemic resides within we rise, rebuild, and tend to what’s between scars are still on the mind, heart and soul through shared stories; we learn to heal and grow. An essential and timely resource, this book offers a comprehensive exploration of post-COVID-19 mental health and emotional wellbeing in the Indian population. This book consists of scientific research stories of post-pandemic recovery in a diverse society. Through well-researched chapters, utilizing both qualitative and Quantitative methods it sheds light on the unique challenges faced by diverse populations, from women and children to college students, defence personnel, and the LGBTQIA+ community. With a scientific analysis of the coping strategies adopted by each group, it provides invaluable insights for professionals, educators, policymakers, and anyone interested in understanding the far-reaching impact of the pandemic. A must-read for anyone committed to research aimed at rediscovering and fostering resilience and mental well-being in the post-pandemic world’.

Dr Shahina Praveen, *Psychotherapist and Author, Germany*

‘A well-documented and much-needed collection of studies on the emotional and behavioural health impacts of COVID-19 in India. The balanced integration of both qualitative and quantitative findings enhanced its relevance’.

Dr Razi Faraz Khan, *Assistant Professor and Head Department of Psychology, Govt. MLB Art’s and Commerce College, Gwalior, Madhya Pradesh*

‘It is good to see that this book addresses the challenges marginalized groups face. It indicates that Indian society’s acceptance level is improving. Indeed, good content’.

Ajinkya Pol, *Assistant Professor, Rizvi Institute of Management Studies and Research, Mumbai*

‘The book lives up to its title by skilfully integrating both qualitative and quantitative studies. The book contains-well-curated chapters covering a wide range of topics’.

Dr Basavarajappa M T, *Assistant Professor, Kodachadri Govt. College, Hosanagara, Karnataka*

'If you're seeking to understand the pandemic's impact on specific populations in India, this book is good source for your academic curiosity. While more studies would have added depth, it's a good effort in exploring the effects of COVID-19'.

Dr Gurvinder Singh, *Assistant Professor, Department of Business Studies, Punjabi University, Patiala*

'The collection of nine chapters on nine different populations is a wonderful idea to make it a beautiful collection. With something for everyone, I am of the view that it is a good resource for social science scholars'.

Ms Shipra Gupta, *Assistant Professor, S.D. College, Bulandshahr, Uttar Pradesh*

'Learning about the extensive psychological impact of the pandemic through this book is quite surprising'.

Ms Seema Kaushik, *Assistant Professor, School of Business Administration, Bhagwan Parshuram Institute, Rohini, Delhi*

'This book presents a blend of qualitative and quantitative studies that examines the psychological health needs of specific populations in India post-COVID-19. The book offers a nuanced understanding of the pandemic's diverse psychological impacts. The detailed findings and analysis make it a good resource for researchers, and mental health professionals who are in the process of unearthing the challenges faced by vulnerable communities in India. A good read for those committed to advancing mental health care in post-pandemic contexts'.

Prof Varun Dutt, *MS, PhD, Dean, Resource Generation and Alumni Relations, Associate Professor, School of Computing and Electrical Engineering, Indian Institute of Technology, Mandi*

'The Present Book is an excellent compilation of valuable and diversified chapters on Post COVID-19 issues in Psychological Health particularly across India. The divergence and convergence in demographics; types of research; samples; methodologies etc further add value to the analytical as well as scientific body of knowledge in Psychology for Eastern and Western World'.

Prof (Dr) Novrattan Sharma, *Director AIBAS, Amity University, Maharajpur, Gwalior, MP*

'As a practicing psychologist, I appreciate the book's emphasis on understanding various populations' specific mental health needs, which is crucial for developing tailored interventions. This volume's thematic and methodological diversity makes it a comprehensive resource for researchers, practitioners, and policymakers. I am confident that this book will serve as a valuable reference for anyone interested in the intersection of mental health and the societal impact of the pandemic'.

Dr Arun Sangwan, *Sports Psychologist*

'The fear of the unknown from the COVID virus still lingers in the minds of the generation who faced those dreadful days. This volume is a justifiable attempt to document the challenges and ensuing coping mechanisms in one place. I am sure this book will not only provide rich content but will also serve a reminder of the era when the very existence of humanity was at stake'.

Nabendu Paul, *Assistant Professor, IIM Amritsar*

'The idea to address the needs of a specific group of people post-COVID seems remarkable. I think it would have been better if the book could have added more chapters. I suggest the editor go for the sequel of the book to include more such studies'.

Dr Shweta Goel, *Assistant Professor,*
Magadh University, Bodh Gaya, Bihar

'The idea of bringing together research done on diverse populations in one place seemed commendable. For this, I would appreciate the editor'.

Dr R. Shanthi, *Professor, Erode Sengunthar*
Engineering College, Tamil Nadu

'This book is crucial in understanding the profound psychological and emotional impact the pandemic has had on vulnerable groups. Its focus on qualitative and quantitative data offers valuable insights that will help inform mental health interventions and policy improvements in post-pandemic India. This work is timely and essential for addressing the evolving mental health needs of our society'.

Dr Sanjay Kumar, *Associate Professor,*
Department of Psychology, University of Allahabad

'*Mental, Emotional, and Behavioural Health Needs of Specific Populations of India Following COVID-19: Findings from Qualitative and Quantitative Studies* is a timely and insightful exploration of the psychological challenges faced by diverse groups in India in response to COVID-19. Through a blend of quantitative and qualitative research, the book sheds light on the pandemic's mental health impact, offering valuable data, findings, and practical solutions for addressing the urgent needs of specific Indian populations. A must-read for psychologists, sociologists, policymakers, and anyone interested in understanding and improving physical and psychological well-being in a post-pandemic world'.

Derick H. Lindquist, *PhD, Professor and Dean,*
School of Psychology & Counselling,
O.P. Jindal Global University, Haryana

'Though it is interesting to sift through the pages of this volume, the content is great, and most importantly, the selection of different populations is a wonderful idea, however, it would have been more appropriate if more studies on vulnerable populations had been included. I congratulate the editor and authors for their wonderful work'.

Dr Binayak Kumar Dubey, *Assistant Professor (stage III), Department of Physical Education, Banaras Hindu University*

'The book is worth reading and will be a great reference resource. I suggest every library should have it'.

Dr Pran Banjara, *Assistant Professor, National Law University, Jodhpur*

'The present volume is a small attempt to capture the impact of the deadly virus on the Indian population in just a few chapters–a crispy summary'.

Dr Sandeep Dubey, *Assistant Professor, Dyal Singh College, University of Delhi*

'A resource for psychologists, sociologists, and other stake holders, this book contributes significantly to informed discourses on impact of COVID-19 on specific population of India. It is a must-read for anyone seeking to broaden their perspective on mental health in the post-pandemic world'.

Dr Brajesh Kumar, *Professor, School of Management & Commerce, Dev Bhoomi Uttarakhand University*

'The book thoughtfully examines the psychological challenges that emerged during the Corona crisis, providing evidence-based insights and coping strategies. It is a good reference book for all those who are interested in mental health. The executive summary chapter is a unique feature that helps quickly glance at the contents'.

Prof Nishan Singh Deol, *Professor of Physical Education, Punjabi University, Patiala*

Mental, Emotional, and Behavioural Health Needs of Specific Populations following COVID-19 in India

The book *Mental, Emotional, and Behavioural Needs of Specific Populations following COVID-19 in India: Findings from Qualitative and Quantitative Studies* reviews quantitative and qualitative research, conducted during and post-pandemic, on economic, social, psychological, and health factors across diverse, specific populations in India. It studies numerous psychological elements of COVID-19 in the context of recovery, handling, coping, and resilience and offers practical approaches for reproducing results and outcomes.

The book includes predictors of mental well-being across women survivors, students, migrant women, and neurodivergent populations. Chapters focus on a wide range of themes including the mental health of Border Security Force personnel during COVID-19 and issues of women's violence and mental health problems amongst poor and migrant workers after COVID-19. The book also throws light on sensitive and beneficial topics such as experiences of a mother of an autistic child and the strengthening of LGBTQIA+ mental health through personal growth initiatives.

It is valuable reading for researchers, mental health practitioners, policymakers, and educators to learn about the most recent developments, concerns, and real-world difficulties encountered, and solutions taken in the mental health field following COVID-19, as well as offering implementable methods for replication.

Rajesh Verma is an assistant professor of psychology at Feroze Gandhi Memorial Government College Adampur, Haryana. He is an Air veteran, academic gold medallist, and completed his doctorate from MD University, Rohtak. His area of interest lies in indigenous psychology, cognitive psychology, social psychology, psychometrics, applied statistics organising academic events, and content writing. He is tech-savvy, uploads psychology curriculum content-specific videos, and writes blogs regularly. He loves to interact with students.

Mental, Emotional, and Behavioural Health Needs of Specific Populations following COVID-19 in India

Findings from Qualitative and Quantitative Studies

Edited by Rajesh Verma

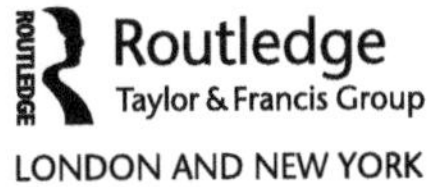

First published 2025
by Routledge
4 Park Square, Milton Park, Abingdon, Oxon OX14 4RN

and by Routledge
605 Third Avenue, New York, NY 10158

Routledge is an imprint of the Taylor & Francis Group, an informa business

British Library Cataloguing-in-Publication Data
A catalogue record for this book is available from the British Library

ISBN: 9781032833682 (hbk)
ISBN: 9781032852485 (pbk)
ISBN: 9781003517313 (ebk)

DOI: 10.4324/9781003517313

Typeset in Times New Roman
by Newgen Publishing UK

मां

and

The Spirit of Humanity!

Contents

Illustrations

Figures

Tables

About the Editor

Rajesh Verma is an assistant professor and student of psychology at Feroze Gandhi Memorial Government College Adampur, Haryana, India. He is an Air veteran, academic gold medallist, and completed his doctorate from MD University, Rohtak. His area of interest lies in indigenous psychology, health psychology, cognitive psychology, social psychology, psychometrics, organising academic events, and content writing. He loves to interact with students.

Contributors

Yogesh Kumar Arya is a professor at the Department of Psychology, Banaras Hindu University, Varanasi. He has completed his PhD in psychology at Banaras Hindu University. He is actively engaged in teaching and research in health and wellbeing, cognition, neuropsychology, and forensic psychology. Dr Arya is currently associated with three research projects awarded by the Education Research and Innovation Council (ERIC), NCERT, New Delhi, UGC and DBT, India. Dr Arya has published more than two dozen research papers and book chapters. He has conducted several workshops on research methodologies and has organised several national and international conferences.

Deepti Aswal is a researcher with a master's degree in applied psychology and a specialisation in social psychology. With a keen interest in qualitative research, she focuses on exploring gender and sexuality dynamics as well as the mental health of children and youth. She aims to contribute to the well-being of individuals and communities through her work.

A. A. S. Azam is currently serving as an assistant professor at Amity University Haryana. With a PhD from Aligarh Muslim University, he has dedicated over 13 years to advancing the field of psychology through rigorous research and teaching. His work emphasises the importance of protective home and school environments in fostering adolescent resilience and published research articles in national and international journals. His roles extend beyond academia, as he is actively involved in mentoring students, coordinating PhD programmes, and guiding interns in counselling and psychological first aid. His passion for integrating technology into education drives his interest in IoT, ICT tools, and mobile app-based mental health interventions. He is an avid reader.

Banani Basistha is an IoE Postdoctoral Research Fellow specialising in Indian Psychology at the University of Hyderabad. She also holds the position of Assistant Editor for the *INSPA Journal of Applied and School Psychology*. Dr Basistha earned her PhD in psychology from Gauhati University, Assam, and brings over eight years of experience in psychological research and teaching. Her contributions to the field are noteworthy, with numerous research articles published in prestigious national and international journals and over 15 papers presented at national and international seminars and conferences. During her research internship at the Indian Statistical Institute (ISI) in Kolkata, she developed a scale to measure and promote pro-environmental behaviour. Her primary areas of interest include Indian psychology, the Indian Knowledge System (IKS), positive psychology, social psychology, health psychology, and organisational psychology.

Vaidya Leena S Bavadekar holds an MPhil in ayurveda and is presently a PhD Scholar. She has worked as an ayurveda physician, consultant, and researcher in Pune for over three decades, focusing on Panchakarma, women's health issues, and lifestyle disorders. She delivered invited lectures to ayurveda students, research scholars, and practitioners at various colleges and institutes on national and international platforms and delivered more than 20 radio talks. Authored over 100 articles in ayurveda journals and newspapers and contributed to *Science India* magazine, published by VijnanaBharati, a prominent Swadeshi science movement. Published books titled *Decoding Leshokta from Ayurveda Samhita (LeshoktaVistar)* and *Ayurveda Panake*. She holds a social responsibility as a 'National General Secretary' of SHAKTI, a national movement for women, working for women's social, cultural, economic, and intellectual empowerment through science and technology. She is involved in social interventions like lectures and interactive sessions highlighting social, physical, nutritional, behavioural, and psychological health concerns for adolescents.

Divya Bhanot is an assistant professor at the Department of Applied Psychology, Ramanujan College, University of Delhi. Dr Bhanot holds a PhD from the University of Delhi. She has constructed the famous Multidimensional Scale of Socio-Political Empowerment. Dr Bhanot has recently received a Grant of $100 from the International Association of Cross-Cultural Psychology and was an awardee by the Asian Association of Social Psychology for 'AASP 2021 Summer School: Best Research Proposal' (2021). She has over ten publications in international journals. Her core research interests lie in the area of applied social psychology.

Benkat Krishna Bharti is an assistant professor of applied psychology at Vivekanand College, University of Delhi. He earned a PhD in psychology from Banaras Hindu University. He has published research papers and presented his research at national and international conferences, seminars, and symposiums. Dr Bharti has resolved to continue working in the academic field for personal growth and excellence, as well as to act creatively and develop core competencies for intrinsically rewarding assignments.

Kangkan Bhuyan is an assistant professor in the Department of English at Chatia College, Assam. He earned his MPhil in American literature from Assam University, Silchar, in 2015, followed by a PhD in 2020, focusing on the exploration of Third Space in postcolonial Indian English literature. Dr Bhuyan currently serves as the Assistant Editor (Content) for the *INSPA Journal of Applied and School Psychology*. He has extensively published in national and international journals and presented his work at international conferences. His dedication to academic excellence was recognised in 2024 when he was awarded the 'Best Academic Coordinator' for the North-Eastern Region by the ICT Academy, Chennai. Passionate about literature, philosophy, and psychology, Dr Bhuyan is committed to fostering a research-oriented mindset among students. His core areas of interest are IKS, health and well-being, American literature, Indian English literature, and postcolonial literature.

Kiran Chaudhary is a distinguished medical professional, with a PhD from JNU, serving as Consultant, Transfusion Medicine at ABVIMS & Dr R.M.L. Hospital in New Delhi. She is known for her innovative approaches to improving patient outcomes and ensuring the highest standards of quality and safety in blood transfusion services. As a member of the Technical Resource Group, a National advisory body, she regularly contributes to policy making. Her contributions to medical education extend beyond the hospital. She has presented several papers at national and international conferences. Throughout her career, Dr Kiran Chaudhary has received numerous awards and fellowships—notable ones being WHO and Harold Gunson Fellowships.

Sreeja Das is working as an assistant professor at Amity University Rajasthan, Jaipur. She earned her doctorate in psychology from BHU. She has published numerous articles in national and international journals. She has an NLP certification and works as a school counsellor in Delhi. She specialises in neuropsychology, clinical psychology, and forensic psychology.

Aishwarya Jaiswal is a senior research analyst at Mercer Mettl. She has been a University Grants Commission Senior Research Fellow in Psychology. She is an awardee of two BHU Gold Medals, prestigious endowment scholarships, and numerous academic and research awards. She is also among the 40 international early career researchers selected from across the globe for the prestigious 'Emerging Psychologist Programme 2021+' organised by the International Union of Psychological Sciences (IUPsyS) and the International Congress of Psychology (ICP). Besides, she received a prestigious bursary award from the British Psychological Society.

Harleen Kaur is a doctoral candidate and ICSSR Junior Research Fellow in the Department of Psychology at Banaras Hindu University. She is a former Indian Youth Delegate from the Ministry of Youth Affairs and Sports, India. She has won prestigious endowment scholarships and numerous academic and research awards. She is also a former Ministry of Social Defence and Social Justice intern. She has several high-impact factor publications in various esteemed international journals. Her areas of interest are gender, social, health, and cognitive psychology.

Pradnya Nitin Kulkarni is an assistant professor at Sir Parashuramabhau College, Pune, Maharashtra. For over 20 years, she has worked as a postgraduation faculty in clinical psychology, counselling psychology, and school psychology. She is a faculty member and coordinator for SWYAM MOOC courses, 'Counselling Psychology' and 'Psychological Disorders'. She has published national and international research papers and book chapters in the domains of health psychology, clinical psychology, positive psychology, and school psychology. She is a trainer in mental health and positive psychology and has experience in counselling for children, youths, and women.

Ketoki Mazumdar, Assistant Professor of Psychology at FLAME University, Pune, is a leading scholar with a PhD from the Tata Institute of Social Sciences, Mumbai. With a decade of experience in teaching and counselling, her research focuses on the intersections of gender, mental health, clinical and cross-cultural psychology, and self-compassion. Dr Mazumdar has significantly contributed to the field with several publications and has led three major national research projects funded by prominent organisations such as ICSSR-New Delhi, TISS-Mumbai, and APA. Her expertise enriches her teaching, as she integrates cutting-edge research into her curriculum, enhancing the learning experience for her students. Passionate about reading and storytelling, Dr Mazumdar continues to inspire and mentor students while exploring real-life struggles and redemptions.

Udisha Merwal has an undergraduate degree from the University of Delhi in Applied Psychology. She researched 'peace of mind' and secured the best undergraduate research paper award. Currently, she works as a public accounting assistant in Canada while pursuing her Post-Baccalaureate Diploma in Accounting from Thompson Rivers University.

Shalini Mittal completed her PhD in psychology at Banaras Hindu University. She works as an assistant professor at the School of Liberal Arts, Bennett University, India. She is trained in the skill of interviewing victims of crime and aims to amplify the voices and impact of victims, gender, and minorities through her research work.

Sonali Mukherjee is working as an assistant professor in the Department of Psychology, School of Humanities and Social Sciences, CHRIST (Deemed to be University), Delhi NCR. Her areas of interest are cognitive psychology, child psychology, clinical psychology, and counselling, and she has more than eight years of work experience. She has researched several topics like neurodevelopmental disorders, specifically dyslexia and autism. She is a certified Neuro-Linguistic Programming (Level 1 and 2) Practitioner by Mind Masters Organisation. She has been a DRDO fellow. Besides that, she has received the best paper presentation award at an international conference. She has published and guided many research papers and major and minor research projects. Currently, she is guiding two PhD scholars. She is a member of a professional body, i.e., IAAP. Currently, she is engaged in several projects related to socioemotional learning, the imposter phenomenon, and the development of ICT tools for dyslexic children.

Swati Pathak has been actively involved in developing the curriculum for certificate courses at Montfort College, Bangalore, and CHRIST (Deemed to be University), Delhi NCR. She had over nine years of experience in counselling and education. She is associated with various organisations that work with child and women's welfare. She has participated in more than 30 national and international conferences/seminars and workshops and presented research papers. She has also been awarded the best paper presentation at an international conference organised by AIIMS, Delhi. Her areas of interest include family and relationship counselling, adolescent counselling, psycho-oncology, and health psychology.

Raosaheb Raut is a PhD candidate who serves as an assistant professor at NMIMS Deemed to be University, Mumbai. Formerly an assistant professor at the Department of Applied Psychology and Counselling Centre, University of Mumbai, he has published extensively in national and international journals. Raosaheb's interest primarily lies in qualitative research and suicide-related behaviour, and he is committed to deepening comprehension in these pivotal areas, striving to effectuate meaningful change through his research endeavours.

Shefalika Sahai is a registered clinical psychologist presently working at Even Healthcare, Bengaluru. She holds an MPhil in clinical psychology from Dr Ram Manohar Lohia Hospital, with First Rank. Her experience ranges from working with adults, adolescents, and children to dealing with issues such as anxiety, mood disorders, behavioural addictions, psychological problems stemming from medical conditions, stress-related problems, and relationship issues. Her research on 'Impact of parental cancer on family dynamics of adolescents' earned her the Best Paper award at the Post Graduate Student Conference on Interdisciplinary Research in Inclusive Growth, Christ University, Bengaluru, in 2015.

Swathy Sathyapal is a PhD candidate in psychology at the Department of Liberal Arts, Indian Institute of Technology Hyderabad. She is also a University Grants Commission Senior Research Fellow. Her PhD work utilises quantitative and qualitative methods to explore the influence of sociocultural attitudes towards appearance on individuals' well-being in the Indian context, including the effect of sociodemographic identities. Before this, she earned her master's degree in applied psychology from Pondicherry Central University. Her other research interests include critical psychology, gender and well-being, women's mental health, body image studies, and family dynamics in Indian culture. Swathy prioritises contextualising her work to the Indian scenario using a culturally sensitive lens. She has presented her research at multiple national and international conferences.

Fouzia A. Shaikh is currently affiliated with Amity University Haryana, India, as a full-time assistant professor. She was awarded with PhD in applied psychology from the University of Calcutta. She has been a recipient of a Junior Research Fellowship and Senior Research Fellowship at the Indian Statistical Institute

(ISI), Kolkata, from 2006 to 2011 after having qualified for all India level Junior Research Fellowship Entrance Examination conducted by ISI, Kolkata. During her doctoral research, she also received an IBM Travel Grant and ISI, Kolkata International Conference Participation Travel Grant in the year 2010 for conference participation in Paris. In the same year, she was invited by the Department of Health Psychology, Free University, Berlin, as a guest researcher and also to deliver an invited talk on assessment tools for health and addiction research. She had worked as a counselling psychologist for the school sector in Uttar Pradesh and offered consultancy to school-goers, parents, and teachers. She has several publications in national and international journals. She has been an ardent reader, writer, and observer and inclined towards performing and visual arts. As a licensed art therapist, she often indulges herself in creating and appreciating different forms of art by diverse populations and age groups.

Shivantika Sharad is an associate professor of applied psychology at Vivekananda College, University of Delhi. Her doctoral research has been on developing the construct of authenticity and has been well-received. She has eight book chapters and over 20 research publications in international journals. The International Association of Cross-Cultural Psychology has recently awarded her 2023 SPARK research grant. Her areas of interest include self and identity, Indian psychological thought, educational pedagogy, social and cultural psychology, and the psychology of the marginalised and East-West studies. She is also a Conscious Parenting Method TM Certified Coach and has served as a Guest Associate Editor of a research topic in *Frontiers in Pain Research.*

Pragya Sharma is a clinical psychologist and the founder of Psyche in Motion, where she provides teletherapy services to adults and couples worldwide. She holds a doctorate in clinical psychology from AIIMS, New Delhi, and MPhil in clinical psychology from IHBAS. Dr Sharma has been recognised for her contributions to the field, receiving the prestigious Youth Fellowship Award from the World Congress of Psychiatry. She is a member of the American Psychological Association (APA) and a lifetime member of the Indian Association of Clinical Psychologists (IACP), and she is certified by the Rehabilitation Council of India (RCI). Dr Sharma has authored numerous book chapters and papers focusing on depression, OCD, anxiety disorders, and the LGBTQ+ population, to name a few. Her areas of specialisation include depression, anxiety, adjustment issues, stress-related issues, relationship issues, behavioural addiction, self-growth and development, marital/couple therapy, emotional management, motivation, and life transitions.

Vikas Sharma, MSc statistics, is a Lead at Statistical Research & Analysis, Catalyst Clinical Research. He provides statistical leadership and guidance to teams working on clinical research projects across multiple therapeutic areas. He combines both academic and industry experience and has more than six publications in peer-reviewed scientific journals.

Tushar Singh has a DPhil in psychology from the University of Allahabad and served as an assistant professor at Banaras Hindu University, India. His research focuses on understanding the miseries of and advocating for the rights of gender and social minorities, including but not limited to LGBTQ+, abused women and children. He has many publications in national and international journals. He has numerous professional recognitions, including the 'Emerging Psychologist' award from the International Congress of Psychology in South Africa in 2012 and the Young Researcher Award by the International Council of Psychologists in Montreal, Canada, in 2018. Dr Singh is a member of the editorial committees of several reputed journals. Currently, he is serving as president (elect) of the National Academy of Psychology, India, and as a member of the board of directors of the International Association of Applied Psychology (IAAP).

Bhawna Tushir is an assistant professor of psychology at Christ University, Delhi-NCR, India, with extensive experience in Malviyan and Gandhian Philosophy. She has worked with several universities and organisations as a trainer and consultant. She is committed to providing rigorous and evidence-based research, ensuring that the findings are reliable and contribute to the existing knowledge in the field.

Soumya T Varghese is an assistant professor at the Jindal Institute of Behavioural Sciences (JIBS), O. P. Jindal Global University. She received her PhD in psychology from the Vellore Institute of Technology, Chennai. Her primary area of interest revolves around academic performance, focusing on identifying and facilitating factors that contribute to it. NCERT, Government of India, funded her doctoral research. Throughout her career, she has taught various subjects, including research methods, educational psychology, organisational psychology, and mental health at both undergraduate and postgraduate levels.

Rahul Varma completed his PhD from BHU, specialising in cognitive psychology, social psychology, personality, and cyberpsychology. With numerous research publications and book chapters in national and international journals, Dr Rahul has demonstrated a solid commitment to advancing the field of psychology.

Sunil K. Verma is currently working as an Associate Professor at Vivekananda College, Delhi University, India. He has published over 50 research papers in reputed national and international journals and has published book chapters in applied social psychology, social gerontology, and family research. Besides this, he has authored a book entitled 'Family. Dynamics and Intergenerational Relations: Psycho-Social Analysis'. He has participated in various national and international conferences. He was the Principal Investigator of multiple projects, including Suicide in Sikkim: A Psycho-Social Study, A Psycho-Social Study on Intergenerational Relation in Interdependent Society, and The Grass is Not Always Greener on the Other Side: A Study on Male Marginalisation and Victimisation. Dr Verma has received several fellowships to participate in international conferences from UGC Travel Grant, IUPSY, and ARTS. In 2012, Dr Verma was selected as an Emergent Psychologist in Cape Town by IUPSY and ICP 2012.

Rudra Vijhani is currently pursuing a bachelor's with Honors at Amity University, Haryana. Rudra has a keen interest in Indian psychology, child psychology, and life span development, which aligns with his academic pursuits and internships in clinical and child psychology. He has actively contributed to the university community by heading the Animal Welfare Department of the YUVA Club, where he developed content for the department, and co-headed the First Responders Team at Artemis Foundation in Hyderabad. As the Sports Coordinator of the Psychology Department, Rudra led the team to its first victory in the inter-sports competition since the establishment of the campus. Beyond academics, Rudra enjoys reading scriptures, playing basketball, and conducting research, reflecting a well-rounded personality with a balance of intellectual and physical interests.

Vineetha K J is an assistant professor of psychology at Markaz Arts and Science College, affiliated with the University of Calicut. She holds a PhD from Mahatma Gandhi University. She was employed as a research assistant at the Inter-University Centre for Disability Studies, Mahatma Gandhi University. With her extensive experience as a counsellor, she has made significant contributions to psychology, providing support and guidance to those in need. Her holistic approach to education ensures that learners develop practical skills for their future careers.

Foreword

Rajesh Verma's edited volume, *Mental, Emotional, and Behavioural Health Needs of the Specific Population Following COVID-19 in India: Findings from Qualitative and Quantitative Studies*, effectively encapsulates the primary theme and issues addressed in the book. I empathise with the individual who has lost all family members; the editor's portrayal of the circumstances in the introduction moved me to tears. I admire his ability to surmount challenges.

This book emphasises the challenges faced by several marginalised groups, including asexual individuals, adults, married women, menopausal women, emerging adults, LGBTQIA+ individuals, students, and domestic workers. The content includes one chapter for Border Security Force (BSF) members, five chapters for women, two for individuals with diverse sexual orientations, one for children, one for emerging adults, and one for students. Forty-five per cent of research focuses on women, indicating that this demographic may be the most adversely affected by the COVID-19 pandemic and need more support, as the impact on women has been greater than on men. This is due to the predominance of female participants in the studies, comprising 45% of the sample.

The selections in this book originated from many regions of India, including North-East India and Kerala, which intensified my curiosity. It piqued my interest. The chapters are systematically arranged, indicating the editor's expertise in the field.

COVID-19 was so horrible that it could destroy everyone who was in its way. India is a microcosm facing numerous issues, particularly due to its population density. The COVID-19 pandemic not only inflicted physical pain but also severely affected the psychological, emotional, and behavioural well-being of the Indian populace. Considering the case's circumstances, it was essential to address the frequently neglected difficulties faced by a certain demographic. One of the content's most commendable attributes is its endeavour to meet the novel demands arising from the new normal.

The integration of quantitative and qualitative research approaches enhances the volume's relevance. Moreover, it is important to acknowledge that the investigations in question extended over an extended duration, specifically during and after the COVID-19 epidemic. The comparative and analytical capabilities afforded by temporal disparities are invaluable. This may facilitate future planning by assessing the magnitude and kind of impact along a temporal continuum.

The chapters of the book mostly address the enduring detrimental psychological repercussions. They are challenging to eliminate; hence, the client and their associates must manage them as required. A notable quality of the book is its examination of many therapies that could have assisted individuals in overcoming their challenges. This book may be highly beneficial for students, researchers, academics, and educators seeking to further their academic careers. It was released recently. Individuals seeking to comprehend the ramifications of COVID-19 may find this volume's findings advantageous.

This volume on one of the most devastating pandemics of the new millennium illustrates the resilience, optimism, and perseverance of the human spirit. It is my sincere hope that it will serve as a scholarly resource that aids in the ongoing efforts of humanity to recover and provide insights for future planning.

Girishwar Misra
Ex-Vice Chancellor, Mahatma Gandhi Antarrashtriya
Hindi Vishwavidyalaya, Wardha and
Former Professor and Head, Department of Psychology,
University of Delhi, Delhi

Preface

The global upheaval caused by COVID-19 shattered a million dreams. And I was witness to one of the shattered dreams.

> It's all over for me; all that I had has been snatched from me. You know, now I am no more than a dead and dry stump. I do not understand how long I will carry this body, a shredded garment. All desires, wants, and needs are dried up, and I am realising that gradually I am becoming emotionless and responseless.

These are a few selected phrases gleaned from a conversation between me and one of my friends just after the second wave of COVID-19. He lost five family members out of a total of six. The ever-smiling man still wears the typical smile, but it lacks the mandatory crowfoot at the end of the eyes. In the evening, when I reclined and my hard mattress caressed my back, I could do nothing except think about the type of thinking my friend might be going through. Immediately, I was reminded of Victor Frankel's book *Man's Search for Meaning*, where he mentions the results of a poll conducted in France, where 89 per cent of participants admitted that what man needs is 'something' for the sake of which he has to live. I suppose my friend has lost that 'something'. In such a continuation of the chain of thoughts, the thought of compiling the requirements of different types of people following the deadly march of the virus crossed my mind and this volume was born. I owe the origin of this volume to my friend.

COVID-19 made the world confront not only physical death and loss but also the indelible impact it had on, the psychological domain. It deteriorated the mental, emotional, and behavioural well-being of all, irrespective of whether they were infected, spared, or working as caregivers. India is the home of almost 18 per cent of the world's human beings. Seeing the scale of population density, COVID-19 had thought of the free run, but thanks to the Govt. of India and the indomitable strength of its people, COVID-19 could not succeed in its sinister designs. As the country grappled with the aftermath of the COVID-19-led pandemic, it became increasingly apparent that addressing the unique needs of specific population groups was essential for future preparedness and complete recovery.

The edited volume, *Mental, Emotional, and Behavioural Health Needs of Specific Population following COVID-19 in India: Findings from Quantitative and Qualitative Research*, is likely to shed light on the multifaceted dimensions of post-pandemic well-being. The combination of quantitative and qualitative is a nuanced approach that seems to be appropriate and is expected to offer a comprehensive exploration of the diverse impact and subsequent manifestation of post-COVID-19 psycho-physical well-being. This volume traverses across India, capturing the essence of the COVID-19-led crisis that unfolded in the Indian population. The notable impact areas that are addressed in the volume include behavioural issues and mental health consequences on children with neurodevelopmental disorders, lived experiences of asexual class, defence mechanisms and loneliness of students, challenges of female domestic workers, resilience among adversity, self-compassion and emotional regulation of working professionals, experiences of mothers of autistic children, and behavioural and health needs of young urban adults. Each chapter examines the specific aspect of the during and post-COVID-19 impact on mental health, drawing on empirical evidence and real-world experiences.

In presenting this collection to the world, I extend my heartfelt gratitude to the contributors whose expertise and dedication have made this volume possible. Their tireless efforts have enriched my understanding of the complex intersections between health, society, and human resilience. The insights gained from the findings underscore the collective commitment towards addressing the mental, emotional, and behavioural health needs of humanity in the wake of COVID-19. I hope that though small some information contained in these pages serves as initiators for better understanding, igniting conversations and initiatives that catalyse in understanding the importance of mental well-being which is a cornerstone of public health across the globe. It is a collective resolve to build a healthier, more resilient future for generations to come.

Rajesh Verma

Acknowledgement

When a project culminates, it gives relief and a sense of satisfaction that I have done what was expected of me by others and by myself. When this volume came to its logical end, I felt for a moment that I had done it. Immediately at the next moment, I suddenly realised that it was not *Me* but rather it was *We* who had done it. I paused for a moment, I couldn't help but burst into laughter at the sheer ridiculousness of my own thoughts. This realisation made me bow my head as a mark of gratitude to all who contributed to shaping this book.

At the outset, I am indebted to all contributing authors who worked tirelessly for so long to provide enriching content for this book. I express my heartfelt gratitude for their efforts and commitment to sharing insightful studies that address the mental, emotional and behavioural health needs of the specific population of India, post-COVID-19.

I express my deepest gratitude to our publisher for believing in me and the significance of this work and for supporting us throughout the publication process. Your guidance and professionalism have been instrumental in shaping this book.

My heartfelt thanks to my dedicated peer reviewers who provided valuable feedback and constructive criticism, helping me refine and improve the content, making it more comprehensive and meaningful.

I thank all coronavirus warriors who managed the pandemic efficiently and circumvented the larger damage which could have devastating effects. Your dedication was unparalleled and will be remembered for a long time to come.

I am thankful to our families and friends for providing total support during this endeavour without expecting reciprocal support from our side.

I am immensely grateful to Dr Uzaina and Dr Sujit Verma (my wife) for their unstinted support, guidance and cooperation in shaping these pages. You both are wonderful human beings who are no less than a storehouse of genuine motivation for me.

Lastly, I thank all those wonderful people who will sift through this volume and further enrich the literature to better understand and create sustainable preparedness paradigms for coming generations.

Thank you, everyone, for your invaluable contributions to *Mental, Emotional, and Behavioural Health Needs of Specific Populations following COVID-19 in India: Findings from Quantitative and Qualitative Research*. I am truly grateful for the opportunity to present this work to the world.

Rajesh Verma

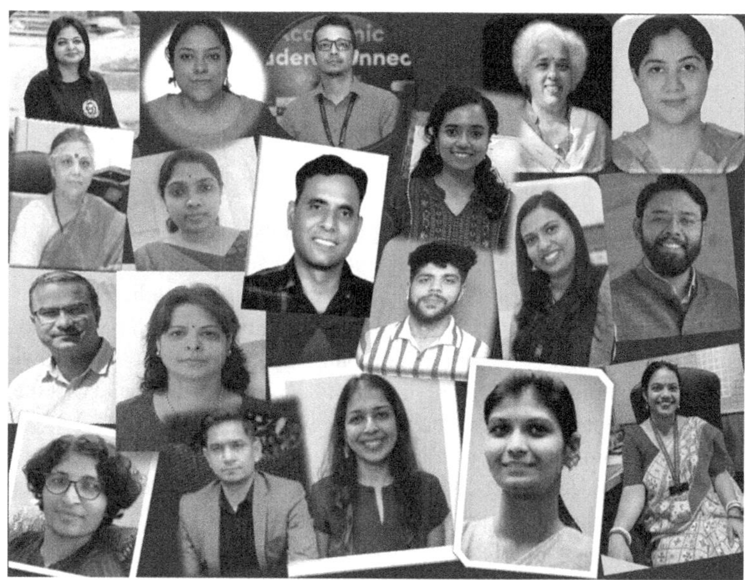

Introduction

Rajesh Verma

Then, why we chose this title? Let me share a brief anecdote. The other day, out of curiosity, I shared the volume's details with a colleague from a different discipline. Upon reading the title, he responded with some optimistic-frowning type facial expressions. He said that why didn't you replace first three words of your title just with 'psychological', to make it concise? At first, his idea seemed valid to me. I was momentarily perplexed and took some time to respond. For others, other than psychology, mental and psychological words are same except they differ on some consonants and vowels. Though unsuccessful, but I tried full throttle to make my colleague understand the nuanced difference with numerous technicalities. This experience made me realise that if a teacher struggles to differentiate between the terms, it would be even more challenging for a novice student.

The 'mental', 'emotional', and 'behavioural' are conceptual dimensions of psychology. The 'mental' dimension is akin to '*manas*' in Sanskrit, where both encompasses major cognitive functions such as thought, perception, and intellect (Thirunavurakasu et al., 2011). Emotional dimension consists of feeling part of affect, while behavioural dimension consists of observable part. Psychology as a whole is a vast field of study that flows between the two banks of science and social science. Heeding my colleague's advice would have been a herculean task, as the current volume already employs a Mixed Method Approach (MMA) to accommodate both qualitative and quantitative studies. Additional burden would have rendered the volume huge and impractical, given the sear size of India and its diversity. Hence, these three words in the title.

A lot has been said and written about the COVID-19 and its impact. However, in comparison to the size of the viral invasion and its distressing effects and after effects, still the literature on post-pandemic psychological is minimal. Interestingly, the literature has addressed almost all issues such as policy and technological interventions history, clinical features, origin, and transmission (Shereen et al., 2020; Sifuentes-Rodríguez & Palacios-Reyes, 2020), psychological impact on varied population (Arora et al., 2020; Das, 2020; Grover et al., 2020), suicide and suicide ideation (Goyal et al., 2020; Mamun et al., 2020; Lee, 2020), epidemiology (Dhar & Oommen, 2020), effect on healthcare workers (Chakma et al., 2021; Chatterjee et al., 2021; Grover et al., 2021; Sunil et al., 2021), coping mechanisms

DOI: 10.4324/9781003517313-1

employed to meet the pandemic led challenges (Barron et al., 2021;Ghosh et al., 2020; Sharma, 2022; Verma, 2024) to name a few concerning the COVID-19. The citations and mentions are not exhaustive; countless other studies have been conducted globally on various aspects of COVID-19. Notwithstanding the availability of COVID-19-related literature, there was a perceived need to compile studies focused on specific populations in India. A specific population refers to a group of people sharing common characteristics such as age, gender, profession, geographical location, mental health problems, specific identities, academics, and marital status. Each population type encountered unique challenges and varied needs from the psychological, social, and physiological perspective during and post-pandemic. Additionally, India is home to the 1.4 billion people with diverse cultures, religions, habits, languages, climatic conditions, ethnicity, and geography, and all have their own stories to share where pandemic impacts are more pronounced than others. Interesting to note that Indians responded to the coronavirus in as diverse a way as the culture of India is. While the virus physically affected everyone similarly, its psychological impact varied from person to person. Consequently, people's needs were as varied as India's culture. This diversity is very unique because that the disease was the same but the ways to deal with it were different and almost all of them proved to be effective. And, this volume is a modest effort to explore and elucidate the multifaceted experiences that addressed the diverse needs, effects, and coping strategies of specific populations during the challenging period through well-adaptive MMA.

MMA was chosen for the following five reasons:

1 Assessment of COVID-19 through single approach would have been an one-sided story, hence qualitative and quantitative studies complement each other and provide holistic understanding.
2 The pandemic had both measurable and immeasurable effects on people's lives, making it essential to incorporate lived experiences, personal narratives, and the levels and intensity of stress and anxiety faced by specific populations to capture the complete human experience in one volume.
3 MMA includes both subjective and objective analysis which caters to the diversified audience.
4 MMA ensured richness of data that portrays human experiences in more credible and robust forms.
5 MMA offered richer, valid, comprehensive, and practical insights into the effects and impacts of COVID-19.

The edited collection comprises nine meticulously researched chapters, over and above the 'Introduction' and 'Executive Summary'. Each chapter caters to specific population offering insights into the nuanced ways the pandemic has influenced their mental, emotional, and behavioural health. The present endeavour sheds light upon the experiences of asexual individuals, Border Security Force personnel, married women, undergraduate students, women survivors, women domestic workers, emerging adults, LGBTQIA+ and heterosexual individuals, and parents of children with autism. By addressing these diverse groups, the volume seeks to capture the breadth and depth of the pandemic's impact across different segments of society.

The qualitative studies reveal the insights in which the pandemic has affected their daily lives, relationships, family bonding, studies, and psycho-social well-being. For instance, the chapters on asexual individuals highlight how isolation and disrupted daily routines have intensified feelings of marginalisation. Similarly, the experiences of married women and women domestic workers highlight the challenges of increased domestic responsibilities and care burden. Additionally, mother of child with neurodevelopmental disorders presents insights into the heightened levels of psychological distress faced during the pandemic.

The quantitative studies employ standard statistical methods to analyse data collected from online and offline surveys, telephonic interviews, and face to face data collection. These chapters provide empirical evidence on the prevalence of various psychological issues among the selected population. For example, the chapters examining undergraduate students and women survivors show the impact of pandemic on their life as a whole.

The last chapter provides a through overview of each chapter in the form of executive summary for a quicker academic glance. The executive summary is designed to help convince the reader to select a chapter on self-interest while quickly going through the author's recommendations.

As the editor, I extend my gratitude to the contributing authors whose dedicated efforts have made this volume possible. Their work not only advances our understanding of the mental, emotional, and behavioural health impacts of COVID-19 on specific population but also highlights the resilience and strength of the individuals who have been studied. It is my hope that this book will serve as a valuable resource for all stakeholders in managing and developing strategies for improving mental health in the wake of crisis like COVID-19.

References

Arora, A., Jha, A. K., Alat, P., & Das, S. S. (2020). Understanding coronaphobia. *Asian Journal of Psychiatry, 54*, 102384. https://doi.org/10.1016/j.ajp.2020.102384

Barron, M, E., Singhal, D., Vijayaraghavan, P., Seshadri, S., Smith, E., Dixon, P., Humble, S., Rodgers, J., & Sharma, A. N. (2021). Health anxiety, coping mechanisms and COVID 19: An Indian community sample at week 1 of lockdown. *PloS One, 16*(4), e0250336. https://doi.org/10.1371/journal.pone.0250336

Chakma, T., Thomas, B. E., Kohli, S., Moral, R., Menon, G. R., Periyasamy, M., Venkatesh, U., Kulkarni, R. N., Prusty, R. K., Balu, V., Grover, A., Kishore, J., Viray, M., Venkateswaran, C., Mathew, G., Ketharam, A., Balachandar, R., Singh, P. K., Jakhar, K., Singh, S., … Panda, S. (2021). Psychosocial impact of COVID-19 pandemic on healthcare workers in India & their perceptions on the way forward–A qualitative study. *The Indian Journal of Medical Research, 153*(5&6), 637–648. https://doi.org/10.4103/ijmr.ijmr_2204_21

Chatterjee, S. S., Chakrabarty, M., Banerjee, D., Grover, S., Chatterjee, S. S., & Dan, U. (2021). Stress, sleep and psychological impact in healthcare workers during the early phase of COVID-19 in India: A factor analysis. *Frontiers in Psychology, 12*, 611314. https://doi.org/10.3389/fpsyg.2021.611314

Das, S. (2020). Mental health and psychosocial aspects of COVID-19 in India: The challenges and responses. *Journal of Health Management, 22*(2):197–205. https://doi.org/10.1177/0972063420935544

Dhar Chowdhury, S., & Oommen, A. M. (2020). Epidemiology of COVID-19. *Journal of Digestive Endoscopy, 11*(1), 3–7. https://doi.org/10.1055/s-0040-1712187

Ghosh, A., Nundy, S., & Mallick, T. K. (2020). How India is dealing with COVID-19 pandemic. *Sensors International, 1*, 100021. https://doi.org/10.1016/j.sintl.2020.100021

Goyal, K., Chauhan, P., Chhikara, K., Gupta, P., & Singh, M. P. (2020). Fear of COVID 2019: First suicidal case in India!. *Asian Journal of Psychiatry, 49*, 101989. https://doi.org/10.1016/j.ajp.2020.101989

Grover, S., Mehra, A., Sahoo, S., Avasthi, A., Rao, T. S. S., Vaishnav, M., Dalal, P. K., Saha, G., Singh, O. P., Chakraborty, K., Janardran Reddy, Y. C., Rao, N. P., Tripathi, A., Chadda, R. K., Mishra, K. K., Rao, G. P., Kumar, V., Gautam, S., Sarkar, S., Krishnan, V., … Subramanyam, A. (2021). Evaluation of psychological impact of COVID-19 on healthcare workers. *Indian Journal of Psychiatry, 63*(3), 222–227. https://doi.org/10.4103/indianjpsychiatry.indianjpsychiatry_1129_20

Grover, S., Sahoo, S., Mehra, A., Avasthi, A., Tripathi, A., Subramanyan, A., Pattojoshi, A., Rao, G. P., Saha, G., Mishra, K. K., Chakraborty, K., Rao, N. P., Vaishnav, M., Singh, O. P., Dalal, P. K., Chadda, R. K., Gupta, R., Gautam, S., Sarkar, S., Sathyanarayana Rao, T. S., … Janardran Reddy, Y. C. (2020). Psychological impact of COVID-19 lockdown: An online survey from India. *Indian Journal of Psychiatry, 62*(4), 354–362. https://doi.org/10.4103/psychiatry.IndianJPsychiatry_427_20

Lee, S.A. (2020). Coronavirus Anxiety Scale: A brief mental health screener for COVID-19 related anxiety. *Death Studies, 44*, 393–401. https://doi.org/10.1080/07481187.2020.1748481

Mamun, M. A., Bodrud-Doza, M., & Griffiths, M. D. (2020). Hospital suicide due to non-treatment by healthcare staff fearing COVID-19 infection in Bangladesh? *Asian Journal of Psychiatry, 54*, 102295. https://doi.org/10.1016/j.ajp.2020.102295

Sharma, S. D. (2022). India's fight against the COVID-19 pandemic: Lessons and the way forward. *India Quarterly: A Journal of International Affairs, 78*(1), 9–27. https://doi.org/10.1177/09749284211068470

Shereen, M. A., Khan, S., Kazmi, A., Bashir, N., & Siddique, R. (2020). COVID-19 infection: Origin, transmission, and characteristics of human coronaviruses. *Journal of Advanced Research, 24*, 91–98. https://doi.org/10.1016/j.jare.2020.03.005

Sifuentes-Rodríguez, E., & Palacios-Reyes, D. (2020). COVID-19: The outbreak caused by a new coronavirus. COVID-19: la epidemia causada por un nuevo coronavirus. *Boletin medico del Hospital Infantil de Mexico, 77*(2), 47–53. https://doi.org/10.24875/BMHIM.20000039

Sunil, R., Bhatt, M. T., Bhumika, T. V., Thomas, N., Puranik, A., Chaudhuri, S., & Shwethapriya, R. (2021). Weathering the storm: Psychological impact of COVID-19 pandemic on clinical and nonclinical healthcare workers in India. *Indian Journal of Critical Care Medicine: Peer-Reviewed, Official Publication of Indian Society of Critical Care Medicine, 25*(1), 16–20. https://doi.org/10.5005/jp-journals-10071-23702

Thirunavurakasu, M., Thirunavukarasu, P., & Bhugra, D. (2011). Concepts of mental health: Definitions and challenges. *International Journal of Social Psychiatry*. https://doi.org/10.1177/0020764011422006

Verma, R. (2024). Coronavirus: The dreaded avatar that surprised humanity. In R. Verma, Uzaina, L. S. S. Manickam, T. Singh, & G. Tiwari (Eds), *Exploring the Psycho-Social Impact of COVID-19: Global Perspectives on Behaviour, Interventions and Future Directions* (pp. 1–18). Routledge: New York. www.routledge.com/Exploring-the-Psycho-Social-Impact-of-COVID-19-Global-Perspectives-on-Behaviour/Verma-Uzaina-Manickam-Singh-Tiwari/p/book/9781003357209

1 'At What Point Should I Bring Up My Asexuality?'

Lived Experiences of Asexuals in the Post-Pandemic Era

Deepti Aswal and Raosaheb Raut

Introduction

According to the Asexuality Visibility and Education Network (AVEN, n.d.) – host to the world's largest online asexual community:

> An asexual person does not experience sexual attraction – they are not drawn to people sexually and do not desire to act upon attraction to others in a sexual way. Unlike celibacy, which is a choice to abstain from sexual activity, asexuality is an intrinsic part of who we are, just like other sexual orientations. There is considerable diversity among the asexual community in the needs and experiences often associated with sexuality including relationships, attraction, and arousal.
>
> (AVEN, n.d.)

As a sexuality, asexuality began to enter the global discourse following two publications: (1) an academic paper on human asexuality, where 1 per cent of a British national probability sample identified as asexual (Bogaert, 2004), and (2) a media report interviewing David Jay, founder of AVEN (Westphal, 2004). Yet, statistics on the global asexual population remain questionable. While the most commonly cited figure is that of 1 per cent of the world population (Bogaert, 2004), a more recent American survey revealed that 4 per cent of individuals aged 18–24, and 1 per cent of the individuals aged 35 and above identify as asexual (Gay and Lesbian Alliance Against Defamation (GLAAD, 2017)). That asexuality can easily blend in within the heteronormative majority – is a chief reason for sparse research on the asexual population (Cottais, 2021).

A key development is the categorisation of asexuality as being placed along a continuum or a spectrum of asexual identities (Scherrer, 2008), due to the growing realisation of a distinction between sexual and romantic attraction. Fundamental to this distinction is the Split Attraction model, primarily given by the asexual and aromantic communities on AVEN (Loggins, 2022); it postulates that while most people are *parioriented*, i.e., their sexual orientation matches their romantic orientation (e.g., a bi person is both bisexual and biromantic), few people are *varioriented*: their sexual and romantic orientations do not match (e.g., romantic

DOI: 10.4324/9781003517313-2

asexual people). Additionally, it is also possible to have a sexual orientation different from one's romantic orientation (e.g., homoromantic and asexual) (Cottais, 2021).

It is crucial to understand how the challenges asexuals face differ from those faced by other LGBTQIA+ identities. Opposition towards same-sex marriage is usually explicitly based on the supposed sanctity of man–woman marriage (Chasin, 2014). However, the biggest argument against asexuality, i.e., sexual normativity, materialises in more inconspicuous contexts, often justified as being vocalised out of concern: suggestions of asexual people 'missing out' on sex or 'labelling' themselves as asexual too soon (Chasin, 2014). Przybylo (2011) coined the term 'sexusociety' to depict the integration of sexuality and society, which surmises (hetero)sexuality to be the norm, thus disparaging all non-sexual relationships (Przybylo, 2011, as cited in Chasin, 2014). This disseminates the belief that not wanting sex means that there is something wrong with the person. Indeed, attempts to underline the causes of asexuality have often resulted in its categorisation as a pathology: as an extreme variant of Hypoactive Sexual Desire Disorder, and/or Female Sexual Interest/Arousal Disorder (American Psychiatric Association, 2013; Gressgard, 2012).

Furthermore, the invalidation experienced by self-identified asexuals may stem not just from the heteronormative society, but also from within the LGBTQIA+ community. As explained by J. Decker, author of *The Invisible Orientation: An Introduction to Asexuality*, inclusion or exclusion within the LGBTQIA+ umbrella is often based on the amount of oppression members of a community face from the larger society. Many queer people believe that whatever discrimination asexuals face cannot amount to that experienced by other groups (such as gays, lesbians, trans-persons), asexuality should not be included within the LGBTQIA+ community (Decker, 2015). Consequently, the LGBTQIA+ community, which is a safe haven for its many members to seek acceptance, might just be another source of rejection for people on the asexual spectrum.

Asexuals may also face a multitude of hurdles in negotiating their identity in romantic relationships. Romantic asexuals (asexuals who experience romantic attraction towards others), who want to pursue relationships with other people may face multiple difficulties, especially when entering a relationship with a non-asexual individual, e.g., negotiating their sexual orientation, preferred level of physical intimacy, etc. (Bogaert, 2015). In a highly sexualised dominant culture, where 'everybody is out for sex', attempts to explain one's lack of sexual attraction may result in ridicule of identity and rejection, often compounding the stigma and marginalisation experienced by asexuals (Sumerau et al., 2018). Studies on the mental health of the asexual population reveal that in comparison to their non-asexual peers, asexual youth have a greater likelihood of reporting a host of mental health concerns, such as higher self-perceived stress as well as higher depressive, anxious, and somatic symptoms (Borgogna et al., 2019; Yule et al., 2013). Additionally, internalisation of the societal delegitimisation of asexuality and the interpersonal stigma experienced by asexual youth may aggravate their asexual identity development (McInroy et al., 2020).

The process of identity development, which is guided by both cultural and societal factors, acts as a key determinant of wellbeing, especially for non-heterosexual populations (Misra, 2007; Thoits, 2013). For sexual-minority individuals, sexual identity development, which involves the cognitive and emotional comprehension of an individual's sexuality (involving sexual attraction, desires, behaviours, values, and relationships, etc.) can present dual opportunities: for exploration and self-discovery, or being inhibited or contrived (Kelleher et al., 2022; Morgan, 2013; Torkelson, 2012). Cass' (1979) theory of Sexual Identity Formation is one of the most prominent models of identity development among non-heterosexual individuals; it posits that as the non-heterosexual individual becomes cognisant of one's sexuality, identity development process entails questioning: exploring the emerging identity and engaging in non-heterosexual related social and sexual activities (Cass, 1979; Kelleher et al., 2022).

However, evidence suggests that sexual identity development doesn't necessarily follow a similar trajectory for asexual individuals. Robbins et al. (2015) proposed an identity development model involving experiences unique to asexual individuals. Due to a lack of informational resources, many asexuals tend to question the validity of their asexuality and even pathologise their lack of sexual attraction. Furthermore, discovering an asexual identity is regarded as a unique process: asexual individuals usually gain information via online resources and communities specific to asexuality (Kelleher et al., 2022). Finally, disclosing one's asexuality is considered to be a crucial component for attaining external validation, as well as the opportunity to educate others, which facilitates identity integration (Robbins et al., 2015; Kelleher et al., 2022). A more recent study (Kelleher & Murphy, 2022) which explored identity development among asexual women also showed similar findings: an awareness of the self-being distinct from the mainstream society initiated the development of participants' asexual identity, which was greatly supported by external resources such as the online asexual community (Keller & Murphy, 2022). Studies show that during the pandemic, the disrupted routine offered a unique opportunity for many queer individuals to explore and build upon their identities, aided by the internet: for it provided LGBTQIA+ resources and community, aiding individuals to understand themselves and connect with similar others (Penfold et al., 2024).

In modern society, nearly all the media portrayal of love and romance is centred on attaining the 'happily ever after': falling in love, getting married, and having children; there is no mention of sexual desires or relationships. The Indian masses are so busy trying to influence people's sexual impulses that they have virtually no room left for people who might not experience sexual attraction at all (Anusuya, 2017). Asexuals in India, while experiencing pathologisation and invalidation like asexuals globally, may also face a unique set of challenges. However, modern Indian society considers public sexual expression a taboo. The institution of marriage legitimises sexual expression to fulfil the obligation of creating a family. While many asexuals do want to build a family and/or get married, the validation of sex through marriage leaves asexuals in a hopeless situation (Asexuality: The Indian Perspective, n.d.). The asexual community continues to be greatly ignored by researchers and the public alike in India; the few pitiful references are either associated with celibacy (Srivastava, 2019) or accompanied by gender stereotypes: while females are considered relatively 'asexual' and passive, males are 'sexual' and active.

In the wake of the COVID-19 pandemic, research endeavours are being made to highlight the challenges faced by the various communities under the LGBTQIA+ umbrella: social disconnectedness due to the lockdown, deteriorating mental health, inequality in accessing healthcare, uncertainty regarding social rituals (such as Pride celebrations), as well as experiences surrounding the 'new normal' in a post-pandemic era (Banerjee & Nair, 2020; Banerjee & Rao, 2021; Bhalla & Agarwal, 2021). Despite these research endeavours, asexuality continues to be a relatively understudied phenomenon in Indian society. This may further compound the challenges asexuals face while navigating through their identity. Thus, the present study was conceptualised to explore the lived experiences of Indian individuals who themselves identify as asexual, or as a part of the asexual spectrum of identities, with the following research questions:

- How do asexuals arrive at acceptance of their asexual identity?
- What are the various forms of challenges faced by asexuals?
- How do asexuals deal with the challenges that they face?
- How do various local psycho-social factors shape their mental health?

Method

Participants

The criteria for inclusion in the study were:

1. individuals aged 18 and above,
2. who self-identified as asexual or as a part of the asexual spectrum, and
3. lives in India.

Using purposive convenience sampling, eight individuals were recruited to participate in the study. On eventual follow-up, two volunteering participants dropped out of the study, bringing the total number of participants to six. The six participants were individually interviewed, and their demographic details have been listed in Table 1.1. Each participant was provided with an identification code (e.g., Participant 1 is P1) to ensure confidentiality of their identity.

Procedure

Online methodologies often offer larger access to populations that are marginalised and less visible in offline contexts, particularly the LGBTQIA+ communities (Riggle et al., 2005). As such, messages about the study were posted on social media platforms to recruit study participants. A semi-structured interview guide

Table 1.1 Demographic details of the participants

Participant	*Age*	*Sex*	*City of Residence*	*Employment Status*	*Relationship Status*
P1	21	Female	Indore	Student	Single
P2	34	Female	Bangalore	Employed	Single
P3	23	Female	Chennai	Employed	Single
P4	28	Female	Mumbai	Employed	Single
P5	29	Female	Bangalore	Employed	Single
P6	23	Female	Pune	Student	In a relationship

(see Appendix) was developed based on the specified research questions, and aimed to capture detailed descriptions of the participants' experiences surrounding their asexuality: realisation of asexual identity, interpersonal relationships, challenges faced in navigating asexual identity, and various local psychosocial factors related to one's mental health. For each (individual) interview, probes were asked as needed to elicit richer responses. Three experts were consulted to review the guiding questions. Based on their feedback, the questions were refined to finalise the interview schedule. After obtaining informed consent, and assuring confidentiality of responses and identity, individual interviews were conducted with the six participants primarily in English. The interviews lasted between 45 and 65 min and were conducted via Zoom meetings to allow recording of the discussion. Verbal consent was taken for recording the interviews, to transcribe the discussions for analysis.

Data Analysis

The data (transcribed manually) were analysed using Interpretative Phenomenological Analysis (IPA), a qualitative approach that utilises the fundamental principles of phenomenology, idiography, and hermeneutics to understand how people make sense of their personal and social worlds, and the meanings they assign to particular events and experiences (Smith & Osborn, 2003). IPA views the participants as experts who can provide a first-hand perspective on the phenomenon being studied (Larkin et al., 2006). Furthermore, IPA's flexible methodology is appropriately fitting to investigate phenomena of the various categories under the LGBTQIA+ umbrella (Chan & Farmer, 2017).

The first stage of analysis involved a thorough reading of each transcript – several times – to develop exploratory comments focusing on the semantic content of the transcript. This led to assigning of initial codes, to reduce the volume of details, while maintaining the complexity (Smith & Osborn, 2003). The codes thus created were clustered together to develop emergent themes, grouping similar themes to form superordinate themes. This series of steps was carried out for each of the six interview transcripts. Following this, the researcher studied the themes and looked for patterns emerging across interviews. Atlas.ti (Licence: L-AFB-F6F) software was utilised to aid data coding and analysis.

Results

Using the IPA approach, seven superordinate themes were identified from the transcripts, which have been listed in Table 1.2.

Coming to an Asexual Identity

Theme 1 explains four subordinate themes (Table 1.2). For most participants, acceptance of asexual identity emerged after a lot of struggle; it began with the realisation that they felt a 'lack' of something (akin to a sense of emptiness) others around them were experiencing. This led to efforts to fit in, to prove themselves as 'normal'.

Table 1.2 List of superordinate and subordinate themes

Superordinate and subordinate themes
Coming to an asexual identity
Experiencing a lack of something
Attempts to fit in
Acceptance of asexual identity
Coming out experience
Selective disclosure
Negative reception of asexual identity
Invalidation from the queer community
Positive responses to coming out
Navigating through romantic relationships
Negative experiences with dating apps
Being invalidated by partner
Dating anxiety
Disturbances in mental health
Exhaustion
Hopelessness
Isolation
Self- doubt
Coping with invalidations
Drawing boundaries
Seeking therapy
Role of online spaces
Asexuality and the Indian Society

Experiencing a Lack of Something

For most participants, recognition of asexual identity began with the realisation that everyone around them was experiencing something about dating and sexual attraction, which they were not. They began understanding that while sex plays an important role in most people's lives, it wasn't the case for them.

> I didn't realise that sexual attraction can be so strong; the extent of how much I don't feel it, how much it doesn't affect my life – until I thought about it.
>
> (P1)

Attempts to Fit In

For participants 4 and 5, the realisation of being different from others brought along attempts to 'fit in', i.e., trying to force themselves to date and/or have crushes, even though they weren't comfortable.

> I think I kind of forced myself to have crushes, because that was what was expected, what was normal.
>
> (P4)

A desire to avoid feeling out of place, coupled with societal and peer expectations fuelled this behaviour on the participants' end. This held especially true for P4 and P5, who are both in their late 20s: at the 'right' age to find a partner and get married (according to societal norms).

Acceptance of Asexual Identity

Acceptance of asexual identity came about in diverse ways for each participant. P3, for instance, knew she wasn't heterosexual, but was unaware of the term 'asexual'.

> I eventually started to know what each letter stood for in LGBTQIA+; that's when I got to know about asexuality; I felt at home, that this really had a name.
>
> (P3)

For P4 and P5, contrarily, the road to acceptance wasn't quite so smooth. They stated that there was a long time – accompanied by a lot of struggle – before coming across the term 'asexual' and accepting that it applied to them or that they identified with it

Coming Out Experience

Theme 2 (Table 1.2) sheds light on the participants' experiences surrounding the disclosure of their asexual identity to others. While disclosure was generally met with negativity, some people did accept participants' asexuality. Most participants preferred coming out to only their close friends and siblings.

Selective Disclosure

All participants have come out to, and prefer discussing their asexuality, with a select few individuals in their personal life, which includes their closest friends, and siblings for some participants. The reason for both is primarily the trust and comfort they share in those relationships, which provided the participants with confidence that would be accepted.

> I mean, we have been very close for a very long time. So, I think I expected them to be okay with everything.
>
> (P3)

Contrary to this, none of the participants have even thought about opening up about their sexuality to their families, consequently for fear of being rejected and misunderstood.

Negative Reception of Asexual Identity

On coming out, most participants were subjected to stereotypes such as 'not having met the right person', 'being in a phase', and having their identity dismissed, or worse, pathologised. On the other hand, the invalidations P6 faced when she came out as greysexual (also known as grey-asexual, referring to an individual who experiences limited sexual attraction, i.e., very rarely or with very low intensity) were rooted in her sexual history.

> A lot of people invalidated it. Because of my past, because I've hooked up with many people, it was like "How can you be asexual?"
>
> (P6)

(*greysexual refers to an individual who experiences limited sexual attraction, i.e., very rarely or with very low intensity)

This may point to the lack of understanding of asexuality being placed along a spectrum, and not being a unitary identity.

Invalidation from the Queer Community

Two participants also faced invalidations from members of queer community; which was astonishing to them, as they expected the queer community to be broad-minded and accepting of identities that lie outside the heteronormative norm.

> I met this guy who was thinking he might be nonbinary. He's that liberal, but he still could not wrap his head around asexuality. He said, "Maybe you just haven't met the right person; maybe you're into girls?"
>
> (P4)

Astonishingly, P2 was subjected to the pathologisation of her greysexuality by a demisexual person (an individual who feels sexual attraction towards someone only after they've developed a strong emotional bond with them), i.e., another member of the asexual community.

> Someone demisexual thought I had to get help because I was greysexual when I told them that my attraction might change for the very same person … So this person told me I should seek a sex therapist for my condition.
>
> (P2)

Positive Response to Coming Out

Amid an overall negative reception to identity disclosure, some participants did find respite in the form of acceptance from select loved ones, who simply accepted the participants' asexuality.

> All she was trying to do was be there for me. I think she didn't really ask a lot of questions, because she just wanted to understand things from my perspective.
>
> (P2)

Navigating through Romantic Relationships

Theme 3 (Table 1.1) explains four subordinate themes which focus on how attempts at dating and building romantic relationships also brought about distressing experiences for some participants. While some dealt with offensive questions on dating apps, others had their asexuality invalidated by their partner.

Negative Experiences with Dating Apps

Some participants recounted the unpleasant things they had to deal with while foraying into the online dating scenario. It appears that most people believe that being on a dating app naturally alludes to the person being interested in sex; those who defy this notion are met with disbelief. Under the guise of curiosity, people don't hesitate to break propriety and ask all sorts of intrusive, offensive questions.

> Other things people were curious about was if I masturbate, or if I kiss people-all of those very personal things.
>
> P1

Being Invalidated by Partner

Some participants recounted hurtful experiences where they had their asexual identity invalidated by their partners at the time. These experiences had a long-lasting impact on the participants. For P2, who was in her first serious relationship, feelings of hurt were masked by anger at her partner for falsely claiming that they understood greysexuality when they did not.

> Even our break up was because I was asexual. That was the most difficult thing, as someone did not understand how my attraction works as a grey-asexual person.
>
> (P2)

Dating Anxiety

For some participants, attempts at dating were accompanied by bouts of anxiety. This indicates how dating can be a nerve-wracking experience for an asexual, especially concerning opening up about their asexual identity with a partner, and negotiating said identity in the relationship.

> I was literally reading up on Reddit, dating advice-stuff like that. It was like, oh, I'm meeting someone tomorrow; let me look at the forums to see what to expect, how to behave, what to communicate, all of that.
>
> (P5)

Disturbances in Mental Health

In response to the question of if (and how) the harrowing experiences had any effect on the participants' mental health, a variety of disturbances came to light. Constantly justifying one's sexuality can be exhausting, often accompanied by feelings of hopelessness and isolation, at being treated as not a part of the 'normal' society.

Exhaustion

Most participants agreed that while having to constantly field interrogations and backlash regarding one's asexual identity is frustrating to no end, it also takes a toll on their emotional wellbeing. After a point, exhaustion seeps in.

> It's difficult – to always keep engaging in such a deep, meaningful conversation; it's emotionally and mentally taxing and you can't keep doing it.
>
> (P6)

Hopelessness

While it is the cold reality, feelings of hopelessness creep in when one understands just how deeply embedded the notion of sex and sexuality is in the world they inhabit.

> When I was newly trying to date, I was not expecting these reactions from people … I felt a bit hurt and disappointed. Hopeless too, because it meant that unless sex was on the table, people were probably not going to want to date me.
>
> (P2)

Isolation

As P4 explained, being continually exposed to the notion that asexuality holds no place in society for it defies societal norms leads to an asexual person being excluded from mainstream society. This makes for an isolated existence and causes one to retreat into a shell for fear of further invalidations.

> I think a part of it is also the isolation, when everyone is making it seem like the biggest thing in life is finding a soulmate and sex is the greatest thing. And if you feel differently, it is very isolating. I think having people say things and try to convince you that you're not that (asexual), just makes you feel more isolated.
>
> (P4)

Coping with Invalidations

Theme 5 (Table 1.1) discusses the coping mechanisms participants use to deal with the distressing experiences they have had to encounter. Two major strategies emerged – (i) drawing boundaries to protect oneself, and (ii) the role played by therapy.

Drawing Boundaries

Initially, most participants spared no efforts to educate people about asexuality, even answering questions they may be uncomfortable with. However, most people continued to ridicule them. This led to a harsh realisation that some people might never accept them. Consequently, participants now draw strict boundaries, setting a limit on their interactions about their asexuality.

> I don't expect much out of people, so I'm like fine, you don't understand. Why should I bother defending myself when they don't even have the capacity to understand? This is who I am. If you want to really understand me then try reading about it.
>
> (P3)

Seeking Therapy

Three participants have sought therapy as a way to manage the distress arising from consistent invalidations. For some, therapy helped them get accustomed to the fact that some people will always try to delegitimise their identity, but that doesn't mean they are true. For P5 though, therapy played a dual role, in helping her manage her anxiety surrounding relationships, and validating her feelings and struggles.

> So two ways that (therapy) helps- having a sounding board, dealing with my thoughts and feelings; and also her (therapist's) experience comes into making me feel like I'm not the only one tackling these issues.
>
> (P5)

Role of Online Spaces

Almost all participants talked about the integral role that online spaces played in aiding asexual identity development, especially since asexuality often finds no representation in real life. The most notably mentioned online platform was Reddit, which is a host to various asexual communities built for varying purposes (providing information, asking doubts, sharing memes, making friends, etc.); an attractive feature is the provision of complete anonymity to the user.

> I started to do a Google search, and came across a Reddit page that was all about asexuality; so many of my questions got answered because so many people were also asking them. I read about it and became friends with a lot of asexual people.
>
> (P1)

Moreover, online asexual communities also offer the opportunity to meet (and make friends with) people with similar experiences.

> So my current group of friends are people from the community who I met through virtual space. And this is where I found other asexual people. I realised that there are many people like me. The resonance I got from this virtual space, that's when I started talking about my attraction as an asexual person to others.
>
> (P2)

Asexuality and the Indian Society

The final theme has important connotations in the context of this study, for it explored the participants' perceptions about the scenario of asexuality in India. Most participants agreed that given the still low acceptance towards LGBTQIA+ communities in India, recognition of asexuality has a long way to go. One of the participants discussed how the origins of problems for Indian asexuals might differ from those of asexuals in Western cultures.

> When I was in boarding school, sex wasn't that big of a thing at that age, there was not as much pressure as there was on people when I went to America … I think it (expectations of being in a relationship) felt a little more, post-college

> here (India) because that's when you are expected to actually be seeing someone and settling down with them.
>
> (P4)

P2, P4, and P5, all of whom are in their late 20s (and early 30s, for P2) also talked about the stifling expectation of marriage and its centrality in Indian society. The pressures and expectations of marriage act as a major source of distress for asexuals.

> It is a given that I have to get married, considering the familial and societal expectations, and all that. How do I navigate that? When I am talking to a potential match, at what point will this (being asexual) come up? Yeah, it does cause anxiety.
>
> (P5)

Discussion

The present study attempted to explore the experiences of asexuals while navigating through their asexual identity in the Indian context. The creation of a self-image during identity development is presumed to occur through experiences and their connected meanings within one's community (Jamil et al., 2009). As asexual people often find 'no similar others' and no representation, growing up in a heteronormative hypersexualised society where sex is supposed to be a necessary part of life often leads to them feeling as though they are somehow different from the normative society. This awareness often marks the beginning of asexual identity development for most asexuals, as also depicted in the present findings (Kelleher & Murphy, 2022).

The participants attempted to reason out their lack of sexual attraction, even going to the extremes of going on dates despite their discomfort, seeking to demonstrate the magnitude of the importance society places on sexual attraction, and its necessity in the human experience. This again, is a key part of the asexual identity development process (Kelleher & Murphy, 2022). It is here that the role of online spaces becomes integral (Robbins et al., 2015). In the absence of a real-life asexual role model to guide their identity development, online asexual communities offer educational resources and ameliorate the sense of otherness that may exist due to aces being considered as being 'deviant' from societal norms (Kelleher & Murphy, 2022). Research during the pandemic has also highlighted the role played by online spaces in helping individuals explore and build their gender and sexual identities, by acting as an avenue for comparison, validation, and self-understanding (Penfold et al., 2024).

Members of the queer community may also invalidate asexuality (Decker, 2015), as observed in the case of P4. It might be reasoned that for individuals from the LGBTQIA+ community, who have had to fight to achieve the right to express their non-heteronormative sexuality the way they want, the idea of not utilising the fruits of this fight may seem dismissive. Oddly, P2's greysexuality was invalidated by a demisexual individual, a member of the asexual community. It appears that greysexuality, which is difficult to explain due to its seemingly vague nature, is seen as being less valid than demisexuality, which can be more concretely conceptualised. If this holds true, then it might point out to the necessity of the dichotomy of a person's sexuality: either you feel sexual attraction (e.g., a demisexual, for whom sexual attraction is rooted in a strong emotional connection), or you don't feel it (like an asexual). However, with little to no research to back up this statement, it is merely a guided observation.

Studies indicate that while the coming out process for sexual minority individuals is often a stressful experience, it may also advance their personal growth and enhance their self-esteem (Vaughan & Waehler, 2010). That the participants' attempts at coming out were mostly met with a negative reception depicts how asexuals are incessantly subjected to dismissal and pathologisation regarding their identity, while also having to deal with stereotypes –'being in a phase', 'not having met the right person', and so on (Robbins et al., 2015).

The recognition of sex as 'natural' and 'necessary' (Kennon, 2021) may further enhance the invisibility and oppression of asexual individuals (Kelleher et al., 2022). Attempting to negotiate an asexual identity in a society where sex is often considered the most vital part of a relationship can result in distressing experiences – being asked intrusive questions, constantly invalidated and dismissed, subjected to disbelief and offensive remarks, and so on (Van Houdenhove et al., 2014). All these serve to make a person feel irrelevant and isolated, as described by the participants.

Asexual individuals, like other sexual minority individuals, are believed to internalise their existence outside of heteronormative ideals and standard life events (McInroy et al., 2020), which also plays an important role in their identity development process (Kelleher et al., 2022). The experience of social rejection, isolation, and stigmatisation, often resulting from identification as a part of a non-heterosexual minority, can negatively affect an individual's mental wellbeing (Mayer et al., 2014).

Mental health has widely been associated with one's interpersonal connectedness, which involves factors such as social networks, social acceptance, and feelings of belongingness (McCallum & McLaren, 2010). Exhaustion at continuously having to explain one's identity paves the way for a hopeless realisation of how completely unaware most people are about your sexual orientation: something that is so crucial to your identity. It makes for an isolated existence when one faces the harsh realisation that their identity finds no place in the larger society.

High levels of perceived social acceptance and belongingness have been linked to better mental health among non-heterosexuals (Kuyper & Fokkema, 2010), for it appears that sexual minority individuals consider acceptance of their sexuality when evaluating if they are being accepted by others (Bjorkman & Malterud, 2012). As such, identifying as an asexual place oneself in a hopeless situation of either having to hide one's identity or come out and face persistent rejection, both of which make way for loneliness due to an isolated existence; this loneliness is increasingly being associated with mental health concerns (such as depression) among non-heterosexual individuals (Eres et al., 2021).

With regards to how the participants deal with the distressing experiences and combat their mental health consequences, two major mechanisms emerged: drawing boundaries and seeking therapy. In this context, drawing boundaries involves setting limits for self as to the extent to which one will engage with questions regarding one's asexuality. By limiting the degree of answering people's queries, or even disconnecting oneself from a toxic conversation, a person preserves their mental health. It must be noted that this is merely an observation on the researcher's part; the present findings augment further examinations before providing any conclusive explanations. Additionally, therapy has been a preferred coping mechanism against discrimination, as well as an aid in better acceptance and understanding of one's sexual identity (Doan Van et al., 2019).

Finally, two chief points emerged from participants' responses regarding the Indian scenario of asexuality: (i) a complete lack of awareness among the general public, and (ii) the stifling expectation of marriage. These offer a glimpse into certain crucial aspects regarding the Indian asexual experience (at least in urban spaces) while warranting further investigations. Building self-concept in non-Western cultures (including India) involves an interdependent view of self: it often conveys the idea that one's existence is meaningful only when one feels included within the society (Usborne et al., 2010). Even though it has been 4 years since the annulment of Section 377 (which originally criminalised all sexual acts 'against the order of nature', including consensual intercourse between LGBTQIA+ individuals), awareness and acceptance towards LGBTQIA+ communities still have a long way to go in the Indian society (Singh, 2022); understanding asexuality appears to be an even longer journey. The question arises – how are asexuals expected to build a positive self-concept when asexuality is not even acknowledged as a legitimate identity?

Again, given the exploratory nature of the present study, as well as the lack of literature regarding the topic of investigation, the current findings raise more questions than they answer. Only future research examining these specific observations can offer a better insight into the dynamics of asexuality in Indian society.

Limitations and Implications

Like all research endeavours, the present study is not exclusive of any limitations. First, India is a culturally and linguistically diverse country, which may have influenced the participants' asexual experiences in ways the study was unable to capture. Second, asexuality exists along a spectrum of sub-identities (such as demisexuality, greysexuality, and so on); the present study neither differentiated nor addressed the experiences of individuals with these sub-identities or their layered romantic and/or sexual orientations. Additionally, while some participants' experiences with therapy have been explored, the study did not address the specific reason(s) for seeking therapy or distinguish individuals with any pre-existing mental health and/or psychiatric concerns. Moreover, while using social media to recruit participants offered wide access to the asexual community, it did further limit the sample to individuals who are fluent in English and are avid social media users. Further, the sample consists solely of asexual women, whose experiences may differ from those of asexual men.

However, exploration of asexual individuals' experiences, who are often viewed as being 'not normal' solely due to their lack of sexual attraction towards others, goes to depict how integral sex is in constituting the 'normal' experiences in our society. Given the present findings about the lack of awareness about and acceptance of asexuality among the Indian masses (as well as the queer community, as experienced by some participants), asexuals undergo a host of experiences throughout their asexual identity development – from the moment of realisation to their current degree of comprehension and acceptance of their asexual identity. The emotional turmoil they may have to experience due to acephobia highlights the need to educate people about asexuality, to make it a part of the social discourse. By providing a glimpse into the life experiences of Indian asexuals, the present study also attempts to highlight the need to develop a more culturally appropriate model for a (a)sexual identity development. Moreover, understanding how the unique challenges asexuals face affect their mental wellbeing, can inform key elements of counselling practices with asexual clients, and aid in the development of more culturally sensitive therapeutic interventions. Given the limited amount of information available about asexuality in the Indian context, perhaps the chief contribution of the present study may be to raise questions for further investigation through future studies.

Conclusion

The present study is an attempt to explore the lived experiences of individuals who identify as a part of the asexual spectrum. The results highlighted participants' experiences as asexuals in a society full of misconceptions, their narratives about self-acceptance, and struggles with interpersonal relationships amidst a widespread lack of acceptance. Owing to the pervasive notions of sexual normativity, self-acceptance for the participants was preceded by a period of struggle, with the realisation of the self-being 'different' from others. Given the lack of resources available in the sexually normative society, online spaces often play a crucial role in aiding the development of an asexual identity. Societal pressures surrounding marriage and widely prevalent misconceptions surrounding asexuality can make navigating through romantic relationships a distressing experience for asexuals. Persistent invalidations and a general lack of acceptance from both loved ones and the larger society can further deteriorate the mental health of asexuals, contributing to feelings of self-doubt, hopelessness, and isolation.

These findings highlight a need to build a comprehensive understanding of the spectrum of sexuality, to create awareness about asexuality and the struggles experienced by the asexual community. Henceforth, the present study primarily intends to encourage more discussion on asexuality to ensure greater visibility and inclusivity of the asexual community within Indian academia as well as among the Indian masses.

Statements and Declarations

Funding

The authors declare that no funds, grants, or other support were received during the preparation of this manuscript.

Conflict of Interest

The authors declare that they have no conflicts of interest.

Informed Consent

Informed consent was obtained from all participants in the study, and for recording the interviews. To ensure participants' confidentiality as well as anonymity, all identifying information was removed from the transcripts. Each participant was referred to via their identification codes (P1–P6), which have also been used in the method section to describe their demographic details and in the Findings section to identify the source of quotations.

Data Availability

The data that support the findings of this study is available on request from the corresponding author. The data are not publicly available for it contains information that could compromise the privacy of the research participants.

References

American Psychiatric Association. (2013). *Diagnostic and Statistical Manual of Mental Disorders* (5th ed.). Arlington, VA: Author.

Anusuya, S. I. (2017, February 3). *"There's Someone Else Just Like You": Inside India's Asexuality Networks*. GenderIT.org. www.genderit.org/feminist-talk/%E2%80%98there%E2%80%99s-someone-else-just-you%E2%80%99-inside-india%E2%80%99s-asexuality-networks

Asexual Visibility and Education Network (AVEN). (n.d.). *Overview*. www.asexuality.org/?q=overview.html

Asexuality: The Indian perspective. Asexualityindia.org. (n.d.). https://asexualityindia.org/theindianperspective.html.

Banerjee, D., & Nair, V. S. (2020). "The untold side of COVID-19": Struggle and perspectives of sexual minorities. *Journal of Psychosexual Health*, *2*(2), 113–120. https://doi.org/10.1177/2631831820939017

Banerjee, D., & Rao, T. S. S. (2021). "The Greying Minority": Lived experiences and psychosocial challenges of older transgender adults during the COVID-19 pandemic in India, a qualitative exploration. *Frontiers in Psychiatry*, *11*. https://doi.org/10.3389/fpsyt.2020.604472

Bhalla, R., & Agarwal, S. (2021). Life in a pandemic: Intersectional approach exploring experiences of LGBTQ during COVID-19. *International Journal of Spa and Wellness, 4*(1), 1–16. https://doi.org/10.1080/24721735.2021.1880204

Bjorkman, M., & Malterud, K. (2012). Lesbian women coping with challenges of minority stress: A qualitative study. *Scandinavian Journal of Public Health, 40*(3), 239–244. https://doi.org/10.1177/1403494812443608

Bogaert, A. (2015). Asexuality: What it is and why it matters. *The Journal of Sex Research, 52*(4), 362–379. https://doi.org/10.1080/00224499.2015.1015713

Bogaert, A. F. (2004). Asexuality: Prevalence and associated factors in a national probability sample. *Journal of Sex Research, 41*(3), 279–287. https://doi.org/10.1080/0022449040 9552235

Borgogna, N., McDermott, R., Aita, S., & Kridel, M. (2019). Anxiety and depression across gender and sexual minorities: Implications for transgender, gender nonconforming, pansexual, demisexual, asexual, queer, and questioning individuals. *Psychology of Sexual Orientation and Gender Diversity, 6*(1), 54–63. https://doi.org/10.1037/sgd0000306

Cass, V. C. (1979). Homosexual Identity Formation: A theoretical model. *Journal of Homosexuality, 4*(3), 219–235. https://doi.org/10.1300/J082v04n03_01

Chan, C. D., & Farmer, L. B. (2017). Making the case for interpretative phenomenological analysis with LGBTGEQ+ persons and communities. *Journal of LGBT Issues in Counselling, 11*(4), 285–300. https://doi.org/10.1080/15538605.2017.1380558

Chasin, C. D. (2014). Making sense in and of the asexual community: Navigating relationships and identities in a context of resistance. *Journal of Community & Applied Social Psychology, 25*(2), 167–180. https://doi.org/10.1002/casp.2203

Cottais, C. (2021, December 20). *Asexuality: A Sexual Orientation Still Unknown and Pathologised.* Grow Think Tank. www.growthinktank.org/en/asexuality-a-sexual-orie ntation-still-unknown-and-pathologi

Decker, J. S. (2015). *The Invisible Orientation: An Introduction to Asexuality*. Skyhorse Publishing. New York.

Doan Van, E. E., Mereish, E. H., Woulfe, J. M., & Katz-Wise, S. L. (2019). Perceived discrimination, coping mechanisms, and effects on health in bisexual and other non-monosexual adults. *Archives of Sexual Behavior, 48*(1), 159–174. https://doi.org/10.1007/ s10508-018-1254-z

Eres, R., Postolovski, N., Thielking, M., & Lim, M. H. (2021). Loneliness, mental health, and social health indicators in LGBTQIA+ Australians. *The American Journal of Orthopsychiatry, 91*(3), 358–366. https://doi.org/10.1037/ort0000531

GLAAD. (2017). *Accelerating Acceptance 2017: A Harris Poll Survey of Americans' Acceptance of LGBTQ People.* Retrieved fromwww.glaad.org/files/aa/2017_GL AAD_Accelerating_Acceptance.pdf

Gressgård, R. (2012). Asexuality: From pathology to identity and beyond. *Psychology & Sexuality, 4*(2), 179–192. https://doi.org/10.1080/19419899.2013.774166

Jamil, O. B., Harper, G. W., Fernandez, M. I., &Adolescent Trials Network for HIV/AIDS Interventions. (2009). Sexual and ethnic identity development among Gay–Bisexual–Questioning (GBQ) male ethnic minority adolescents. *Cultural Diversity and Ethnic Minority Psychology, 15*(3), 203–214. https://doi.org/10.1037/a0014795

Kelleher, S., & Murphy, M. (2022). The identity development and internalisation of asexual orientation in women: An interpretative phenomenological analysis. *Sexual and Relationship Therapy*, 1–31. https://doi.org/10.1080/14681994.2022.2031960

Kelleher, S., Murphy, M., & Su, X. (2022). Asexual identity development and internalisation: A scoping review of quantitative and qualitative evidence. *Psychology & Sexuality, 14*(1), 45–72. https://doi.org/10.1080/19419899.2022.2057867

Kennon, P. (2021). Asexuality and the potential of young adult literature for disrupting all on normativity. *The International Journal of Young Adult Literature*, *2*(1), 1–24. http://doi.org/10.24877/IJYAL.41

Kuyper, L., & Fokkema, T. (2010). Loneliness among older lesbian, gay, and bisexual adults: The role of minority stress. *Archives of Sexual Behavior*, *39*(5), 1171–1180. https://doi.org/10.1007/s10508-009-9513-7

Larkin, M., Watts, S., & Clifton, E. (2006). Giving voice and making sense in interpretative phenomenological analysis. *Qualitative Research in Psychology*, *3*(2), 102–120. https://doi.org/10.1191/1478088706qp062oa

Loggins, B. (2022, January 29).*What Is the Split Attraction Model?* Verywell Mind. www.verywellmind.com/what-is-the-split-attraction-model-5207380

Mayer, K. H., Garofalo, R., & Makadon, H. J. (2014). Promoting the successful development of sexual and gender minority youths. *American Journal of Public Health, 104*(6), 976–981. https://doi.org/10.2105/AJPH.2014.301876

McCallum, C., & McLaren, S. (2010). Sense of belonging and depressive symptoms among GLB adolescents. *Journal of Homosexuality, 58*(1), 83–96. https://doi.org/10.1080/00918369.2011.533629

McInroy, L., Beaujolais, B., Leung, V., Craig, S., Eaton, A., & Austin, A. (2020). Comparing asexual and non-asexual sexual minority adolescents and young adults: Stressors, suicidality and mental and behavioural health risk outcomes. *Psychology & Sexuality*, 1–17. https://doi.org/10.1080/19419899.2020.1806103

Misra, G. (2007).*Construction of self: A cross-cultural perspective.* Mindscapes, Bangalore, India. 32–44.

Morgan, E. M. (2013). Contemporary issues in sexual orientation and identity development in emerging adulthood. *Emerging Adulthood, 1*(1), 52–66. https://doi.org/10.1177/2167696812469187

Penfold, A., Callaghan, P., & Urry, K. (2024). Online communities and identity: Experiences of LGBTQIA+ emerging adults engaging with LGBTQIA+ online content during the COVID-19 pandemic. *Psychology of Popular Media.* Advance online publication. https://doi.org/10.1037/ppm0000529

Przybylo, E. (2011). Crisis and safety: The asexual in sexusociety. *Sexualities, 14*(4), 444–461. https://doi.org/10.1177/1363460711406461

Riggle, E. D., Rostosky, S. S., & Reedy, C. S. (2005). Online surveys for BGLT research: Issues and techniques. *Journal of Homosexuality*, *49*(2), 1–21. https://doi.org/10.1300/J082v49n02_01

Robbins, N., Low, K., & Query, A. (2015). A qualitative exploration of the "coming out" process for asexual individuals. *Archives of Sexual Behavior, 45*(3), 751–760. https://doi.org/10.1007/s10508-015-0561-x

Scherrer, K. (2008). Coming to an asexual identity: Negotiating identity, negotiating desire. *Sexualities, 11*(5), 621–641. https://doi.org/10.1177/1363460708094269

Singh, R. K. (2022, September 6).*Four Years since Article 377 Annulment, Has Anything Changed for LGBTQ Community?* The Logical Indian. https://thelogicalindian.com/lgbtq/four-years-since-article-377-annulment-by-supreme-court

Smith, J. A., & Osborn, M. (2003). Interpretative phenomenological analysis. In J. A. Smith (Ed.), *Qualitative Psychology: A Practical Guide to Research methods*. Sage Publications, Inc.

Srivastava, M. (2019). *Asexuality in India and Hindu mythology [Blog]*. https://themchblog.wordpress.com/2019/05/09/asexuality-in-india-and-hindu-mythology/

Sumerau, J., Barbee, H., Mathers, L., & Eaton, V. (2018). Exploring the experiences of heterosexual and asexual transgender people. *Social Sciences*, *7*(9), 162. https://doi.org/10.3390/socsci7090162

Thoits, P. A. (2013). Self, identity, stress, and mental health. In C. S. Aneshensel, J. C. Phelan, & A. Bierman (Eds.), *Handbook of the Sociology of Mental Health* (pp. 357–377). Springer Netherlands.

Torkelson, J. (2012). A queer vision of emerging adulthood: Seeing sexuality in the transition to adulthood. *Sexuality Research and Social Policy, 9*(2), 132–142. https://doi.org/10.1007/s13178-011-0078-6

Usborne, E., & Taylor, D. M. (2010). The role of cultural identity clarity for self-concept clarity, self-esteem, and subjective well-being. *Personality & Social Psychology Bulletin, 36*(7), 883–897. https://doi.org/10.1177/0146167210372215

Van Houdenhove, E., Gijs, L., T'Sjoen, G., & Enzlin, P. (2014). Stories about asexuality: A qualitative study on asexual women. *Journal of Sex & Marital Therapy*, *41*(3), 262–281. https://doi.org/10.1080/0092623x.2014.889053

Vaughan, M., & Waehler, C. (2010). Coming out growth: Conceptualizing and measuring stress-related growth associated with coming out to others as a sexual minority. *Journal of Adult Development*, *17*(2), 94–109. https://doi.org/10.1007/s10804-009-9084-9

Westphal, S. P. (2004). *Feature: Glad to be Asexual.* New Scientist. www.newscientist.com/article/dn6533-feature-glad-to-be-asexual/

Yule, M., Brotto, L., & Gorzalka, B. (2013). Mental health and interpersonal functioning in self-identified asexual men and women. *Psychology and Sexuality, 4*(2), 136–151. https://doi.org/10.1080/19419899.2013.774162

Appendix
Guiding Questions for the Semi-Structured Interview

1 Can you describe your experiences as an asexual living in India?
2 When did you realise you were asexual?
   a How did this realisation come about?

3 Have you come out to anyone in your life?
   a Motivation for coming out
   b How did they react?

4 What was going on in your head when they responded to you?
   (prompt: thoughts, feelings)

5 How do you feel discussing your sexuality now?
   a What do these conversations sound like?

6 How do you think asexuality is seen in Indian society?
(prompt: responses to hearing the word 'asexual')

7 Have you ever been in/ faced similar situations/ responses?
   a How did you react?

8 Do you think these situations/ responses have an effect on your mental health?
   a How do you cope with them?

9 Is there something that we haven't discussed, but you would like to share with me?

2 Psychological Impact of Institutional Quarantine on Border Security Force Personnel of India

Pragya Sharma, Shefalika Sahai, Vikas Sharma, and Kiran Chaudhary

Introduction

Indian Border Security Force (BSF) is the world's largest border guarding force with more than 6400 km of borders (Chhabra & Chhabra, 2013). BSF works in callous working conditions including poor infrastructure and lack of minimal amenities. They are away from their families and rough out in tough weather and terrain conditions which puts them at a higher risk for adverse psychological outcomes. Previous studies have reported occupational stress and anxiety in this population emanating from insomnia, being apart from family, and poor communication with seniors among other reasons (Chhabra & Chhabra, 2013). This negatively impacts their physical and mental health (Singh & Alam, 2018).

During the COVID-19 pandemic, BSF in India, apart from their regular duties were involved in enforcing lockdown measures and were working with local and state authorities to ensure compliance with quickly changing COVID-19 protocols. They manned checkpoints and controlled the movement of people in border areas. Due to their increased interaction with possibly infected citizens, BSF personnel were at a higher risk of having contracted the virus. Thus, as a precautionary measure, they were quarantined to prevent the spread of COVID-19 within their colleagues, and the broader community.

Quarantine refers to the segregation of individuals possibly exposed to a contagion to observe if they become ill, thereby reducing the risk of infecting others (HSH & CDC, 2017). When confronted with the unique circumstances of a pandemic, people are vulnerable to a variety of psychological and mental health problems. However, quarantine may exacerbate these concerns, especially in the BSF population who are already at risk because of their nature of work. Depression and anxiety are highly prone to develop and exacerbate when there is a lack of social interaction (Xiao & Wang, 2020). Those subjected to institutional quarantine frequently find it uncomfortable (Rubin & Wessely, 2020).

Psychological impact refers to 'the effect caused by environmental and/or biological factors on an individual's social and/or psychological aspects' (Norhayati et al., 2021, p. 1). Anxiety and depression were among the commonly seen psychological impacts as a result of COVID-19 quarantine (Lai et al., 2020; Zhang et al., 2020). Comparing the psychological outcomes of detained individuals with those

DOI: 10.4324/9781003517313-3

who were not, Sprang and Silman (2013) revealed significantly higher levels of psychological distress and depressive symptoms among those who were quarantined.

Intolerance of uncertainty, a psychological vulnerability factor for fear is defined as 'an individual's dispositional incapacity to endure the aversive response triggered by the perceived absence of salient, key, or sufficient information, and sustained by the associated perception of uncertainty' (Carleton, 2016a, p. 31). Higher degrees of uncertainty intolerance is linked to anxiety-related disorders (Carleton, 2016b).

Five elements associated with stress and anxiety symptoms have been linked to the coronavirus: risk and contamination, concerns about the economic fallout, xenophobia (fear or hatred of foreigners) connected to the coronavirus, compulsive monitoring and reassurance seeking, and traumatic stress symptoms (Doshi et al., 2021). Brooks et al. (2020) discovered the negative psychological impact of quarantine like post-traumatic stress disorder (PTSD), disorientation, and hostility. During the quarantine period, people reported feeling dread, nervousness, despair, and guilt (Desclaux et al., 2017). An analysis of 24 studies on the psychological consequences of quarantine revealed that post-traumatic stress symptoms, bewilderment, and rage were common among the sample. Stressors include a prolonged quarantine period, fear of infection, frustration, lack of resources, not enough information, monetary loss, and stigma (Brooks et al., 2020).

Based on existing literature from previous pandemics like SARS and MERS, where increased levels of distress, depression, and anxiety were observed among those quarantined, the variables related to psychological impact were selected (Brooks et al., 2020; Jeong et al., 2016). Subjective distress refers to the immediate emotional discomfort experienced during quarantine. The isolation, disruption of routine, and fear associated with potential contagion can lead to heightened distress, making this an important variable to measure. Depression, commonly seen to result from prolonged isolation, was also considered vital to examine. For BSF personnel, who are accustomed to active and structured environments, the sudden shift to isolation can increase feelings of helplessness and hopelessness, thereby leading to depressive symptoms. Anxiety was chosen due to the uncertainty and fear that often accompany quarantine. BSF personnel, trained for action and control, might find the lack of control during quarantine particularly anxiety-provoking. Lastly, perceived stress was deemed important as it measures the individual's appraisal of their stress levels during quarantine, providing insight into how they are managing the psychological demands of isolation.

By focusing on the above variables, the study aimed to provide an understanding of the psychological impact of quarantine on BSF personnel.

Rationale

Understanding quarantined persons' experiences is crucial for minimising the adverse effects of isolation on mental health in future. There is minimal research on the compliance, challenges, emotional reactions, and psychological effects of BSF personnel when placed under quarantine. The population being unique in functioning and working style was selected to understand the psychological impact (depression, anxiety, perceived stress, and subjective distress) in the event of pandemic-led stressors they faced, such as isolation, disruption of routines, and concerns for family wellbeing, which could have exacerbated the impact on their mental health.

Objective

The present paper aimed to assess the psychological effects of institutional quarantine on depression, anxiety, perceived stress, and subjective distress of BSF personnel.

Methods

Study design: This cross-sectional observational study was conducted at a BSF Camp after necessary approval was obtained from the BSF and the ethics committee of Dr Ram Manohar Lohia Hospital, New Delhi. Recruitment was carried out over 1 month (July 2020).

Sample

The study utilised a convenience-based sampling technique to recruit participants from the BSF personnel. Within the last 3 months, 250 personnel had been quarantined at a time at this particular facility. For a population of 250, the sample size was calculated using a 95% confidence level ($Z = 1.96$), a 5% margin of error, and an assumed proportion of 0.5 ($p = 0.5$). To account for potential missed or incomplete responses, the sample size was adjusted by assuming a 10% non-response rate and came out to be 169 individuals.

The final sample comprised 176 individuals (172 male) (18–60 years, mean = 37.80 and SD = 9.62) who provided written consent for participation. Around 3% of the participants had studied up to higher secondary or less, 27% up to higher secondary, 36% up to senior secondary, 31% were graduates, and 2% were postgraduate. Amongst the posts held by the participants, 59% were either head constables or constables, 13% were havildar, about 8% were nursing assistants or medics, 9% were assistant superintendents or superintendents, about 3% were inspectors, and 6% were drivers. Out of the participants, 93% were Hindus, 5% were Muslims, and about 2% were in the other category (Jain, Christian, Sikh).

Inclusion and Exclusion Criteria

All individuals of both genders at the particular BSF camp who had been quarantined at the institutional facility and who could read and comprehend either English or Hindi were included in the study. The participants who had no history of any psychiatric illness were included.

Participants who had tested positive for COVID-19 at the time of data collection and/or had been diagnosed with any chronic medical condition were excluded.

Tools

Impact of Event Scale-Revised (IES-R) (Weiss, 2007)

The IES-R is a self-report measure of present subjective distress. It comprises 22 items rated on a Likert scale from 0 to 4. According to Beck et al. (2008), the IES demonstrated a sensitivity ranging from 0.89 to 1.00 and a specificity between 0.78 and 0.94% for diagnosing PTSD.

Beck Depression Inventory (BDI)-II (Beck et al., 1996)

The BDI is a self-report assessment of 21 items which measures depressive symptoms (Beck et al., 1961). The internal consistency of BDI ranges from 0.73 to 0.92 (Beck et al., 1988).

State-Trait Anxiety Inventory (STAI) (Spielberger, 1983)

The STAI is a 40-item measure for trait and state anxiety. Internal consistency of STAI coefficients varied from 0.86 to 0.95, while test–retest reliability coefficients ranged from 0.65 to 0.75 (Lushene et al., 1983).

Perceived Stress Scale (PSS) (Cohen et al., 1983)

Cohen et al. (1983) developed the PSS which is used to measure how stressful life conditions are perceived. Lee (2012) reported an internal consistency of Cronbach α as 0.84 for the overall sample and 0.86 for English respondents.

The investigators conducted a semi-structured qualitative interview. This focused on eliciting information about the satisfaction of individuals with the quarantine facilities, the difficulties faced, their feelings, and feedback or suggestions on how to make the quarantine process easier for them.

Statistical Methods

Data were analysed using SPSS version 21. The socio-demographic characteristics were analysed using descriptive statistics. Shapiro–Wilk test was conducted to test for normality and it was found that data on most variables were not normally distributed. The association between subjective discomfort, depression, anxiety, and perceived stress was examined using the Spearman correlation. Multiple linear regression models were used to evaluate the predictive relationships between perceived stress, subjective discomfort, anxiety, and depression. A thematic analysis was conducted after the interviews were manually transcribed.

Procedure

For data collection, participants were directly approached and briefed in detail about the purpose and significance of the study—their queries and doubts, if any were clarified before they consented to their participation. After obtaining written informed consent, and explaining the process of filling out the questionnaires, each participant completed the set of questionnaires, which included the IES-R, BDI-II, STAI, and PSS. The entire process took approximately about 45 min for each participant. Additionally, the participants were asked to complete a self-report information form about demographics. Data were collected on a one-on-one basis in a private room to ensure a distraction-free environment.

Ethical Considerations

The study was carried out strictly according to the APA code of ethics for psychological research keeping in mind the ethical principles and according to the Helsinki Declaration. The participation was fully voluntary, and confidentiality was assured.

Results

The findings indicate that of the 176 participants, 94% were married and approximately 5% were unmarried. The socio-economic status of participants indicated that 97% belonged to the upper middle socio-economic class, while around 3% belonged to the upper socio-economic class as per classification by Majumder (2021). Table 2.1 shows the descriptive analysis of psycho-social variables.

Table 2.1 Descriptive analysis of psycho-social variables

Variables		*N*	*Percentage*
SES	Upper	5	2.84
	Upper Middle	171	97.15
Marital	Single	9	5.11
	Married	167	94.88
Traumatic events	Yes	2	1.13
	No	174	98.86
Exposure	Vacation	94	53.40
	Transfer	71	40.34
	Contact with positive	11	6.25
Current fear	Not at all	106	60.22
	Small	53	30.11
	Some	15	8.52
	Moderate	2	1.13
Prev COVID-19	Yes	24	13.63
	No	152	86.36

Table 2.2 shows the descriptive analysis results for subjective distress, depression, anxiety, and perceived stress. The mean score for subjective distress suggested that, on average, participants experienced low levels of subjective distress, although the relatively high standard deviation indicates considerable variability in distress levels. Scores on depression were very low across the sample, with minimal variability. Anxiety levels were reported to be moderate to high and were fairly consistent among participants. Scores on perceived stress were low on average, but while some participants experienced very low stress, others reported significantly higher levels.

Table 2.3 shows Shapiro–Wilk Statistics with *p*-values of parameters of depression, anxiety, distress, and perceived stress, which indicates that data were not normally distributed.

Table 2.4 shows the correlations between subjective distress, depression, anxiety, and perceived stress. Results revealed a significant positive correlation between all variables signifying that greater levels of subjective distress are seen with increased levels of depression, anxiety, and perceived stress. Specifically, depression and anxiety

Table 2.2 Descriptive statistics for subjective distress, depression, anxiety, and perceived stress ($n = 176$)

Variables	*Mean*	*Std. Deviation*	*Minimum*	*Maximum*
Subjective Distress	1.227	1.8188	0.0	10.0
Depression	0.392	1.2281	0.0	10.0
Anxiety	40.568	1.9467	40.0	58.0
Perceived Stress	1.233	2.6224	0.0	17.0

Table 2.3 Test of normality

Variables	*Shapiro–Wilk Statistics*	*p-value*
Depression	0.353	<0.0001
State anxiety	0.104	<0.0001
Trait anxiety	0.403	<0.0001
Perceived stress	0.542	<0.0001
Intrusion	0.545	<0.0001
Avoidance	0.360	<0.0001
Hyperarousal	0.592	<0.0001

Table 2.4 Correlation between subjective distress, depression, anxiety, and perceived stress

Variables	*1*	*2*	*3*
Subjective distress (1)	–	–	–
Depression (2)	0.289**	–	–
Anxiety (3)	0.208**	0.269**	–
Perceived stress (4)	0.295**	0.366**	0.511**

** Correlation is significant at the 0.01 level (1-tailed).

were significantly correlated with perceived stress ($\rho = 0.269, p < 0.01$; $\rho = 0.366, p < 0.01$, respectively) indicating that participants with elevated depressive symptoms also experienced more anxiety and perceived stress. A strong positive relationship was observed between anxiety and perceived stress ($\rho = 0.511, p < 0.01$) indicating that individuals who report higher levels of anxiety also perceived greater levels of stress.

Regression Analysis

Multiple regression analysis (Tables 2.5 and 2.6) results concluded that 35.8% of the variance in depression was explained by perceived stress and subjective distress ($F = 48.309, p < 0.000$). Depression was found to be significantly predicted by perceived stress and subjective distress.

Multiple regression analysis (Table 2.6) results concluded that 22.6% of the variance was indicated by the two predictors ($F = 25.306, p < 0.000$). Anxiety was seen to be significantly predicted by perceived stress and subjective distress.

Thematic Analysis

In subsequent interviews, participants reported several challenges during the quarantine period, primarily concerning practical issues. When questioned about the ideal duration of the quarantine period, most participants seemed to be satisfied with the 14 days, believing it was appropriate given its scientific basis. However, seven participants from the group suggested a shorter quarantine period, typically 7–10 days, provided there were no symptoms. One participant felt that there should be no quarantine at all while another suggested a case-by-case approach, wherein quarantine is suggested after enquiring where the person is coming from. Conversely, one participant suggested that the quarantine duration should be extended to 20 days instead, as it takes time for the symptoms to manifest.

Table 2.5 Regression analysis with perceived stress, subjective distress, and depression

Predictor variable	*ß*	*t*	*Sig.*
Perceived stress	0.503	7.770	0.000
Subjective distress	0.196	3.033	0.003

Dependent variable: Depression.

Table 2.6 Regression analysis with perceived stress, subjective distress, and anxiety

Predictor variable	*ß*	*t*	*Sig.*
Perceived stress	0.358	5.035	0.000
Subjective distress	0.215	3.024	0.003

Dependent Variable: Anxiety

Five themes emerged from the analysis which hovered around the problems the participants faced during quarantine. The themes were:

1. Inadequate Hygiene and Sanitation Facilities
   - **Limited toilet facilities**: Participants, especially in buildings where multiple people shared few bathrooms, found it challenging to maintain social distance, which heightened their concerns about health risks.

     > If we are using one bathroom for ten people, how can we keep ourselves safe from infection?

   - **Inadequate sanitisation measures**: Participants felt that the sanitisation of shared utilities like bathrooms and drinking water facilities was insufficient, contributing to the fear of contact and transmission of COVID-19.
   - **Repeated contact with surfaces**: The necessity of touching shared surfaces, particularly for utilities like drinking water, was seen as a health risk, increasing participants' discomfort and concerns.

     > All of us fill drinking water from the same water cooler. It is not possible to sanitise after each water bottle refill.

2. Insufficient utilities and basic amenities
   - **Shortage of water**: Lack of sufficient water was reported by some participants, contributing to feelings of discomfort and making daily activities difficult.
   - **Unsatisfactory food**: Two participants specifically mentioned that the food provided was inadequate, and one participant expressed frustration over the high cost of food at the facility, preferring home quarantine instead.

     > I am spending so much money on the food here and even the quality isn't that great. I could have been eating at home at a much lower cost.

   - **Limited seating options**: A participant expressed the need for additional seating options like chairs, as only the bed was available, adding to the discomfort.

     > There is only a bed to sit on. It would be better to have a chair each. You can't sit on the bed all day long.

   - **Difficulty adjusting to heat**: Several participants struggled with the lack of cooling systems such as air conditioners or coolers, making it difficult to cope with the temperature.

     > How are we supposed to manage in this heat? It is 40 degrees Celsius, reported one of the participants.

3. Lack of access to essentials
   - **Minimal utility provisions:** Two participants felt that the basic utilities were insufficient, leading to dissatisfaction with the overall living conditions.

- **Online delivery issues**: One participant pointed out that only online delivery was available for essentials, and having more regular physical supplies would have been more convenient.

  'Every time I need something, I have to order it online. It would have been helpful to have a store set up with basic essentials', said one of the participants.

4 Desire for recreational and social engagement

- **Recreational activities:** Many participants expressed a strong desire for recreational activities, such as television access and better internet connectivity, to pass the time. The absence of purposeful activities heightened the sense of isolation.

  'We are habitual to staying busy and active. Now, suddenly, we are confined to one room with no one to talk to and no television or other source of entertainment. It becomes difficult to pass the time all day long', said a participant.

- **Restricted outdoor time**: Most participants expressed a desire to have some outdoor time, feeling 'stifled' in their rooms without the opportunity to go outside and engage with their environment, which negatively impacted their wellbeing.

5 Emotional and psychological discomfort

- **Feeling confined and restricted:** The restriction to rooms, with no outdoor access, led to stifling and frustration, suggesting the negative psychological impact of prolonged confinement.
- **Desire for home quarantine:** One participant's preference for home quarantine due to the cost and dissatisfaction with the facility indicates both financial strain and emotional discomfort. 'I would have been happy to spend this time with my family, have the privilege to eat home-cooked food and save some money as well. Instead, I am here, unhappy and spending unnecessarily on basic necessities and mediocre food.'

This thematic analysis highlighted the importance of addressing both physical (e.g., utilities, hygiene) and psychological needs (e.g., recreation, outdoor access) during quarantine to improve wellbeing. Themes such as the loss of usual routines, limited activities, reduced social contact, and usage of shared resources were major stressors. These collectively impacted the psychological health of the participants.

Discussion

This study attempted to evaluate the psychological impact of institutional quarantine on the Indian BSF personnel. The gender ratio of the sample was representative of the general ratio of those employed in the security forces in India (Saleem & Jan, 2019).

The majority of the participants (60%) reported no fear while 30% reported fear to a small extent. Findings suggest that the majority experienced fear during the initial months of the spread i.e., between March and May 2020. Thereafter, as they received news about the wellbeing of their relatives and others recovering from

COVID-19, their fear subsided. A previous Indian study also reported that a large percentage of their participants reported low fear (Rajeshwari, 2017). This study found that high levels of fear were reported by females and healthcare workers; however, both groups were underrepresented in the sample.

Some individual demographics like age (18–40 years), being married, and belonging to upper socio-economic status were linked to better mental health outcomes (Zhao et al., 2020). The relatively young age, high socio-economic status, and the high percentage of married participants in this study could be linked to lower levels of distress, anxiety, and depression. Previous studies reported younger individuals to tend to experience less emotional distress and have better coping mechanisms during stressful situations (Charles & Carstensen, 2010) while Muntaner et al. (2013) emphasised that higher socio-economic status acts as a protective factor against stress and mental health issues. Also, marriage provides a buffer against mental health concerns, by providing emotional stability and a sense of security, reducing stress and enhancing psychological wellbeing (Simon, 2014).

During a later time of the pandemic when the current study was conducted, participants felt confident that by taking the necessary precautions, they could reduce the risks associated with infection. The findings of the present study are supported by the findings of Posen (2016) which indicated that, in contrast to the pandemic's initial peak, stress and fear levels were lower during the remission (lockdown) phase of the disease.

The participants were aware of the potential economic impacts but were not primarily affected by it as their sense of safety came from their relative economic stability. Previous research reported that insecure employment and uncertainties regarding employment lead to anxiety (Yang & Long, 2024).

The findings reported that uncertainty was the norm for them and thus, it was less distressing for them. They were accustomed to operating in uncertain and dangerous situations, where immediate orders had to be followed without prior information. As a result, they were familiar with living in uncertainty, and this aspect of COVID-19 did not affect them as much. The presence of uncertainty within the security forces is well-accepted and known (Rosser, 2019).

Results showed a strong positive correlation among perceived stress, anxiety, and depression. Increased perception of stress has been seen to be linked to anxiety, depression, interpersonal sensitivity, frustration, and powerlessness (Fernández et al., 2020). The association between perceived stress and depression is well-established (Lee & Kim, 2012; Mamo et al., 2012) with perceived control and anxiety being important mediators.

A significant positive correlation was also seen among subjective distress and perceived stress levels, depression, and anxiety indicating higher the subjective distress the participant was experiencing in quarantine, the higher the perceived stress, depression, and anxiety features. Previous studies reported that the participants who experience moderate to severe subjective distress have significantly higher scores of depressive and anxiety symptoms (Wiegner et al., 2015).

Anxiety and depression were found to be predicted by perceived stress and subjective distress. High perceived stress has been linked to anxiety and depression (Shi et al., 2020; Zhang et al., 2020). A recent study with participants of the initial

COVID-19 outbreak in China concluded high perceived stress level was linked to higher intensity of anxiety and depression (Racic et al., 2017).

When asked about the difficulties they faced during the quarantine, the participants highlighted practical concerns such as sharing of resources which couldn't suffice for social distancing norms. The inadequacy of basic supplies during quarantine has been seen as a source of distress and is associated with anxiety and anger (Yan et al., 2021).

Several participants wished there were more recreational activities such as television, and better internet network connectivity so that they could spend time easily. The loss of usual routine, having limited activities to engage in the isolation room, and reduced social contact has been seen to cause stress, boredom, and frustration among those quarantined (Cheng et al., 2020; Jeong et al., 2016).

Findings suggest that interventions aimed at reducing either perceived stress, subjective distress, or anxiety would have a beneficial impact on other variables. For instance, reducing perceived stress may help lower levels of anxiety, depression, and subjective distress. Understanding these relationships is crucial for developing comprehensive mental health strategies for this population.

Conclusion

This study explored the psychological impact of institutional quarantine on BSF personnel in India, with a focus on subjective distress, perceived stress, depression, and anxiety. The findings revealed low levels of psychological distress, including depression and perceived stress, with moderate levels of anxiety. A key insight from this study is the positive correlation between perceived stress, anxiety, and depression, as well as the strong association between subjective distress and these psychological factors. The findings indicate that while BSF soldiers showed resilience—possibly as a result of their extensive training and exposure to high-stress situations—they also displayed anxiety, underscoring the possible long-term consequences of quarantine.

Thematic analysis revealed important stressors that may have added to the psychological strain of the individuals, including interrupted routines, restricted social connection, and limited activities. These pressures are indicative of more general mental health issues that people under institutional quarantine deal with.

Despite the relatively low levels of psychological distress observed, the significant correlations underscore the need for tailored interventions to address the mental health needs of quarantined personnel. Psychological support, structured routines, and stress management interventions should be prioritised to prevent the escalation of anxiety and depression.

Limitations

The majority of our participants were male which limits the generalisation. The study did not assess whether the participants engaged in any preventive behaviours to mitigate the impact of stress. Since the participants in our study were BSF employees, the findings would be valid for similar groups only. As the study was cross-sectional, only the immediate impact of quarantine could be studied.

Acknowledgements

We acknowledge the support of the BSF forces for their cooperation in carrying out this study.

Data Availability

The data supporting this study's findings are available on request from the corresponding author. The data are not publicly available because it contains information that could compromise the privacy of research participants.

References

Beck, A. T., Steer, R. A., & Brown, G. K. (1996). *Manual for the Beck Depression Inventory-II.* San Antonio, TX: Psychological Corporation. https://doi.org/10.1007/978-1-4419-1005-9_441

Beck, A. T., Steer, R. A., & Carbin, M. G. (1988). Psychometric properties of the Beck Depression inventory: twenty-five years of evaluation. *Clinical Psychology Review*, *8*(1), 77–100. https://doi.org/10.1016/0272-7358(88)90050-5

Beck, A. T., Ward, C., Mendelson, M., Mock, J., & Erbaugh, J. (1961). Beck depression inventory (BDI). *Archives of General Psychiatry*, *4*(6), 561–571. https://doi.org/10.1001/archpsyc.1961.01710120031004

Beck, J. G., Grant, D. M., Read, J. P., Clapp, J. D., Coffey, S. F., Miller, L. M., & Palyo, S. A. (2008). The impact of event scale-revised: psychometric properties in a sample of motor vehicle accident survivors. *Journal of Anxiety Disorders*, *22*(2), 187–198. https://doi.org/10.1016/j.janxdis.2007.02.007

Brooks, S. K., Webster, R. K., Smith, L. E., Woodland, L., Wessely, S., Greenberg, N., & Rubin, G. J. (2020). The psychological impact of quarantine and how to reduce it: a rapid review of the evidence. *The Lancet*, *395*(10227), 912–920. DOI: https://doi.org/10.1016/S0140-6736(20)30460-8

Carleton, R. N. (2016a). Into the unknown: a review and synthesis of contemporary models involving uncertainty. *Journal of Anxiety Disorders*, *39*, 30–43. https://doi.org/10.1016/j.janxdis.2016.02.007

Carleton, R. N. (2016b). Fear of the unknown: One fear to rule them all?. *Journal of Anxiety Disorders*, *41*, 5–21. https://doi.org/10.1016/j.janxdis.2016.03.011

Charles, S. T., & Carstensen, L. L. (2010). Social and emotional ageing. *Annual Review of Psychology*, *61*(1), 383–409. http://dx.doi.org/10.1146/annurev.psych.093008.100448

Chhabra, M., & Chhabra, B. (2013). Emotional intelligence and occupational stress: A study of Indian Border Security Force personnel. *Police Practice and Research*, *14*(5), 355–370. http://dx.doi.org/10.1080/15614263.2012.722782

Cheng, H. Y., Jian, S. W., Liu, D. P., Ng, T. C., Huang, W. T., & Lin, H. H. (2020). Contact tracing assessment of COVID-19 transmission dynamics in Taiwan and risk at different exposure periods before and after symptom onset. *JAMA Internal Medicine*, *180*(9), 1156–1163. http://dx.doi.org/10.1001/jamainternmed.2020.2020

Cohen, S., Kamarck, T., & Mermelstein, R. (1983). A global measure of perceived stress. *Journal of Health and Social Behavior*, 385–396. https://psycnet.apa.org/doi/10.2307/2136404

Desclaux, A., Badji, D., Ndione, A. G., & Sow, K. (2017). Accepted monitoring or endured quarantine? Ebola contacts' perceptions in Senegal. *Social Science and Medicine*, *178*, 38–45. http://dx.doi.org/10.1016/j.socscimed.2017.02.009

Doshi, D., Karunakar, P., Sukhabogi, J. R., Prasanna, J. S., & Mahajan, S. V. (2021). Assessing coronavirus fear in the Indian population using the fear of COVID-19 scale. *International Journal of Mental Health and Addiction*, *19*, 2383–2391. http://dx.doi.org/10.1007/s11469-020-00332-x

Fernández, R. S., Crivelli, L., Guimet, N. M., Allegri, R. F., & Pedreira, M. E. (2020). Psychological distress associated with COVID-19 quarantine: latent profile analysis, outcome prediction and mediation analysis. *Journal of Affective Disorders*, *277*, 75–84. http://dx.doi.org/10.1016/j.jad.2020.07.133

Health and Human Services, H. S., & Centers for Disease Control and Prevention (CDC. (2017). Control of communicable diseases. *Federal Register*, *82*(12), 6890–6978.

Jeong, H., Yim, H. W., Song, Y. J., Ki, M., Min, J. A., Cho, J., & Chae, J. H. (2016). Mental health status of people isolated due to Middle East Respiratory Syndrome. *Epidemiology and Health*, *38*, 1–7. http://dx.doi.org/10.4178/epih.e2016048

Lai, J., Ma, S., Wang, Y., Cai, Z., Hu, J., Wei, N., ... & Hu, S. (2020). Factors associated with mental health outcomes among health care workers exposed to coronavirus disease 2019. *JAMA Network Open*, *3*(3), e203976. http://dx.doi.org/10.1001/jamanetworkopen.2020.3976

Lee, E. H. (2012). Review of the psychometric evidence of the perceived stress scale. *Asian Nursing Research*, *6*(4), 121–127. http://dx.doi.org/10.1016/j.anr.2012.08.004

Lee, S. H., & Kim, S. J. (2012). The degree of perceived stress, depression and self-esteem of university students. *Journal of Korean Public Health Nursing*, *26*(3), 453–464. https://doi.org/10.5932/JKPHN.2012.26.3.453

Lushene, R., Vagg, P. R., & Jacobs, G. A. (1983). *Manual for the State-Trait Anxiety Inventory.* Palo Alto, CA: Consulting Psychologists. www.researchgate.net/publication/235361542_Manual_for_the_State-Trait_Anxiety_Inventory_Form_Y1_-_Y2

Majumder, S. (2021). Socioeconomic status scales: Revised Kuppuswamy, BG Prasad, and Udai Pareekh's scale updated for 2021. *Journal of Family Medicine and Primary Care*, *10*(11), 3964–3967. https://doi.org/10.4103/jfmpc.jfmpc_600_21

Mamo, J., Buttigieg, R., Vassallo, D., & Azzopardi, L. (2012). Psychological stress amongst Maltese undergraduate medical students. *International Journal of Collaborative Research on Internal Medicine & Public Health*, *4*(5), 840–849. http://dx.doi.org/www.researchgate.net/publication/266348975_Psychological_Stress_amongst_Maltese_Undergraduate_Medical_Students

Muntaner, C., Ng, E., Vanroelen, C., Christ, S., & Eaton, W. W. (2013). Social stratification, social closure, and social class as determinants of mental health disparities. *Handbook of the Sociology of Mental Health*, 205–227. https://doi.org/10.1007/978-94-007-4276-5_11

Norhayati, M. N., Che Yusof, R., & Azman, M. Y. (2021). Prevalence of psychological impacts on healthcare providers during COVID-19 pandemic in Asia. *International Journal of Environmental Research and Public Health*, *18*(17), 9157. https://doi.org/10.3390/ijerph18179157

Posen, B. R. (2016). Foreword: Military doctrine and the management of uncertainty. *Journal of Strategic Studies*, *39*(2), 159–173. https://doi.org/10.1080/01402390.2015.1115042

Racic, M., Todorovic, R., Ivkovic, N., Masic, S., Joksimovic, B., & Kulic, M. (2017). Self-perceived stress in relation to anxiety, depression and health-related quality of life among health professions students: Across-sectional study from Bosnia and Herzegovina. *Slovenian Journal of Public Health*, *56*(4), 251–259. http://dx.doi.org/10.1515/sjph-2017-0034

Rajeshwari, R. (2017). *Need for Gender Equality in Security Forces.* The Times of India. https://timesofindia.indiatimes.com/blogs/khaki-dairies/need-for-gender-equality-in-security-forces. Accessed June 24, 2020. https://timesofindia.indiatimes.com/blogs/khaki-dairies/need-for-gender-equality-in-security-forces/

Rosser, B. A. (2019). Intolerance of uncertainty as a transdiagnostic mechanism of psychological difficulties: A systematic review of evidence pertaining to causality and temporal precedence. *Cognitive Therapy and Research, 43*(2), 438–463. https://doi.org/10.1007/s10608-018-9964-z

Rubin, G. J., & Wessely, S. (2020). The psychological effects of quarantining a city. *British Medical Journal, 368*, 1–2. https://doi.org/10.1136/bmj.m313

Saleem, S. M., & Jan, S. S. (2019). Modified Kuppuswamy socioeconomic scale updated for the year 2019. *Indian Journal of Forensic Community Medicine, 6*(1), 1–3. https://doi.org/10.18231/2394-6776.2019.0001

Shi, J., Huang, A., Jia, Y., & Yang, X. (2020). Perceived stress and social support influence anxiety symptoms of Chinese family caregivers of community-dwelling older adults: a cross-sectional study. *Psychogeriatrics, 20*(4), 377–384. https://doi.org/10.1111/psyg.12510

Simon, R. W. (2014). Mental health and emotions. *Handbook of the Sociology of Emotions: Volume II*, 429–449.

Singh, J., & Alam, K. (2018). The effect of stress and coping on paramilitary forces personnel's among different ranks of BSF employees (Border Security Force). *IAHRW International Journal of Social Sciences Review, 6*(5), 791–795.

Spielberger, C. D. (1983). *Manual for the State-Trait Anxiety Inventory STAI (form Y)*. Palo Alto, CA: Consulting Psychologists. https://doi.org/10.1007/978-94-007-0753-5_2825

Sprang, G., & Silman, M. (2013). Posttraumatic stress disorder in parents and youth after health-related disasters. *Disaster Medicine and Public Health Preparedness, 7*(1), 105–110. http://dx.doi.org/10.1017/dmp.2013.22

Weiss, D. S. (2007). The impact of event scale: revised. In In J. P. Wilson & C. S. Tang (Eds.), *Cross-Cultural Assessment of Psychological Trauma and PTSD* (pp. 219–238). Boston, MA: Springer US. https://doi.org/10.1007/978-0-387-70990-1_10

Wiegner, L., Hange, D., Björkelund, C., & Ahlborg, G. (2015). Prevalence of perceived stress and associations to symptoms of exhaustion, depression and anxiety in a working age population seeking primary care-an observational study. *BMC Family Practice, 16*, 1–8. http://dx.doi.org/10.1186/s12875-015-0252-7

Xiao, C., & Wang, G. (2020). Mental health work in the context of the COVID-19 pandemic: What progress have we made so far and what is the next step?. *Journal of Psychiatric Research, 129*, 122. http://dx.doi.org/10.1016/j.jpsychires.2020.05.023

Yan, L., Gan, Y., Ding, X., Wu, J., & Duan, H. (2021). The relationship between perceived stress and emotional distress during the COVID-19 outbreak: Effects of boredom proneness and coping style. *Journal of Anxiety Disorders, 77*, 102328. http://dx.doi.org/10.1016/j.janxdis.2020.102328

Yang, T., & Long, X. (2024). Post-COVID-19 challenges for full-time employees in China: Job insecurity, workplace anxiety and work-life conflict. *International Journal of Mental Health Promotion, 26*(9).

Zhang, J., Lu, H., Zeng, H., Zhang, S., Du, Q., Jiang, T., & Du, B. (2020). The differential psychological distress of populations affected by the COVID-19 pandemic. *Brain, Behavior, and Immunity, 87*, 49. http://dx.doi.org/10.1016/j.bbi.2020.04.031

Zhao, H., He, X., Fan, G., Li, L., Huang, Q., Qiu, Q., ... & Xu, H. (2020). COVID-19 infection outbreak increases anxiety level of the general public in China: Involved mechanisms and influencing factors. *Journal of Affective Disorders, 276*, 446–452. http://dx.doi.org/10.1016/j.jad.2020.07.085

Appendix

Socio-Demographic Form

Date of Assessment:

Name:

Age:

Gender: Male/ Female

Education:

Occupation:

Religion:

Income/ month:

SES: Lower/ Lower middle/ Upper Middle/ Upper Domicile: Urban/ Rural

Marital status:

Family structure: Nuclear/ Joint: Children (if any), their ages: Address:

Phone number:

Previous h/o mental illness: Comorbid physical condition:

Other traumatic events prior to quarantine: On treatment (details):

Medicine(s) ongoing: Exposure type:

Date of admission to quarantine: Distance from home:

Qualitative Data Collection

Current Fear of COVID-19

1 Thinking about COVID-19 makes me feel anxious—not at all/small extent/some extent/moderate extent/large extent
2 I feel tense when I think about the threat of COVID-19—not at all/small extent/some extent/moderate extent/large extent
3 I feel quite anxious about the possibility of another outbreak of COVID-19/this outbreak never-ending—not at all/small extent/some extent/moderate extent/large extent

Satisfaction with the Quarantine Facilities

Overall: Very dissatisfied/dissatisfied/neutral/satisfied/very satisfied.
Living conditions: Very dissatisfied/dissatisfied/neutral/satisfied/very satisfied.
Cleanliness: Very dissatisfied/dissatisfied/neutral/satisfied/very satisfied.
Food: Very dissatisfied/dissatisfied/neutral/satisfied/very satisfied.
Supplies: Very dissatisfied/dissatisfied/neutral/satisfied/very satisfied.
Information provided: Very dissatisfied/dissatisfied/neutral/satisfied/very satisfied.
Staff: Very dissatisfied/dissatisfied/neutral/satisfied/very satisfied
Doctor visits: Very dissatisfied/dissatisfied/neutral/satisfied/very satisfied.
Seclusion: Very dissatisfied/dissatisfied/neutral/satisfied/very satisfied.
Opportunity to interact: Very dissatisfied/dissatisfied/neutral/satisfied/very satisfied.
Any Other:

Interview Schedule

What are your thoughts about the:

Duration of quarantine:

Finances:

Stigma:

What are the difficulties you faced/ concerns during quarantine?:

What feelings did you experience during the quarantine?:

Do you have any suggestions on how to make the quarantine process easier?:

3 Impact of COVID-19 and Social Distancing Measures on Married Women

A Qualitative Enquiry

Shalini Mittal, Tushar Singh, Harleen Kaur, Rahul Varma, Sreeja Das, Yogesh Kumar Arya, Sunil K. Verma, Shivantika Sharad, Divya Bhanot, Udisha Merwal, Aishwarya Jaiswal, Benkat Krishna Bharti, and Bhawna Tushir

Introduction

Although the COVID-19 pandemic impacted both men and women, their experiences were markedly different. While both genders faced significant physical and psychological health challenges, women shouldered a disproportionate burden due to increased gender inequalities during the lockdown. With schools and workplaces closed, both working and non-working women found themselves overwhelmed with unending household responsibilities. For working women, the added pressure of work-from-home only compounded these demands. The result of this was a frantic schedule that left women with extraordinarily little time for themselves, resulting in challenges to their mental and physical wellbeing. Despite the increase in family time, the shift to remote work, home-schooling, and confinement negatively impacted women more than men (Czymara et al., 2020). The unequal distribution of family care and household responsibilities has historically placed a disproportionate burden on women; this was exacerbated by the COVID-19 pandemic. In addition to increased responsibilities and consequent health crises, the pandemic also resulted in increased gender-based violence, unequal distribution of caregiving responsibilities to women, and heightened risks of COVID-19 infection and job loss. Although an increased involvement of men in household activities and childcare was noted during the pandemic, women continued to have a major share of these responsibilities. Alon et al. (2020) also highlighted that employed women were disproportionately burdened with domestic responsibilities during the pandemic. Research suggested that women took additional responsibilities during lockdown, including caregiving and household duties (Wenham et al., 2020). This increased their risk of infection, as past research by Lee and Frayan (2008) indicates that more women are in caregiving roles and are thus more susceptible

DOI: 10.4324/9781003517313-4

to infection due to their involvement in these roles. Hjálmsdóttir and Bjarnadóttir (2021) reported that mothers faced increased mental and emotional labour during the pandemic as they were not only managing increased household responsibilities but were also managing their family members' wellbeing. Several other studies also indicated that working mothers spent more time on household work than their paid jobs during the COVID-19 pandemic (Andrew et al., 2020; Carlson et al., 2021; Collins et al., 2021 Craig & Churchill, 2021; Hennekam & Shymko, 2020; Manzo & Minello, 2020; Qian & Fuller, 2020). Although the COVID-19 pandemic significantly impacted both men and women in the workplace, female-dominated industries such as hospitality, tourism, and entertainment were particularly adversely affected. According to Alon et al. (2020), fewer women as compared to men were in telecommuting jobs and thus had very few opportunities to work from home. In some instances, the pandemic also resulted in reduced gender disparities. Studies highlighted instances of role reversals, where mothers took on frontline professional roles while male counterparts became primary caregivers. Therefore, an increase was observed in the participation of males in household and childcare duties. Although the pandemic positively influenced societal norms surrounding gender roles, there was always a disparity in men's share of responsibilities at home when compared to women. For a majority of women, most of the burden was shared by them only (Farré et al., 2021. This situation persisted until the pandemic was effectively controlled and lockdown restrictions were removed.

Additionally, research also shows that stay-at-home orders led to an increase in domestic violence as families spent more time together, potentially causing individuals to act out as offenders (Hodgkinson & Andresen, 2020; Mittal & Singh, 2020; Maji et al., 2022). Hussain et al. (2020) reported that pregnant women faced challenges in travelling and accessing maternity services due to the lockdown, leading to heightened stress, clinical depression, and anxiety (Wang et al., 2020).

The literature presented above indicates that the COVID-19 pandemic created significant difficulties for both working and non-working women, resulting in increased household responsibilities, health-related issues, and adjustment problems. However, only a handful of research was conducted to explore the experiences and transitions of married women during the pandemic. Therefore, the present research was conducted to qualitatively examine the unique experiences of married women in India during the COVID-19 pandemic and the subsequent lockdown. It was felt that understanding the specific experiences of married women during the pandemic would not only provide valuable insights into the shifting gender roles and choices during the pandemic and the associated consequences but also would inform policy and practice decisions for such future crises.

Method

The research was conducted on a convenient sample of 20 married women from northern parts of India between the age group of 25 and 45 years. The participants were contacted telephonically and were explained the purpose of the research. Following this, informed consent to participate in the study and to record the conversation was obtained. The participants were also informed that the information provided to them would be kept strictly confidential. To ensure confidentiality, the participants were assigned codes and their names were not recorded. The telephonic interviews of participants centred around their experiences during the COVID-19 pandemic and the imposed social distancing norms. Sometimes, the researcher had to probe with questions such as 'What was the workload of household chores?' 'Had there been any change from what it was before the lockdown?', and 'To what extent did you receive help from other members of your family?' etc. The participants responded in either Hindi or English and later, all the narratives were transcribed manually in the English language. All the narratives were thematically analysed and then the themes were identified based on the patterns in the data using Braun and Clarke's (2006) six-step method approach of thematic content analysis.

Results

A total of four major themes about the experiences of married women during the COVID-19 pandemic and the period of imposition of the social distancing norms were identified after a thematic content analysis of the narratives. These include 'emotional and psychological impact', 'social impact', 'impact on workload', and 'coping'. Table 3.1 highlights the themes, subthemes, and descriptions as they emerged in the narratives of the participants.

Table 3.1 Major themes and subthemes

S. No.	*Theme*	*Subtheme*	*Descriptors*	*Examples*
1	Psychological and emotional health	Immured	Feelings of being trapped or caged	'For the first few months, we were completely trapped inside the house, not meeting anybody' Respondent 1. 'I have to stay at home, and I am not used to it. So, it is getting a bit difficult'. Respondent 15.
		Ambivalence/ Mixed feelings	Experience of partly positive and partly negative feelings	'I had a very systematic life but suddenly my life has changed. So, though it has not impacted me much, I have mixed feelings. I crave the older times sometimes. Other times it is okay'. Respondent 16.

(*Continued*)

Table 3.1 (Continued)

S. No.	*Theme*	*Subtheme*	*Descriptors*	*Examples*
		Anxiety	Negative feelings of apprehension	'More than the social distancing norms I think it is the pandemic itself that is problematic and risky. It is anxiety-provoking for everyone'. Respondent 10.
2	Social impact	Social isolation	State of complete or near-complete lack of contact between an individual and society.	'I would say that social life has been ruined completely. We cannot go out to meet friends or family'. Respondent 6. 'Social life has come to a standstill for me'. Respondent 4.
		Emotional intimacy	Increased emotional closeness or improved emotional bonding	'I got married just two years back. With work, I never got much time with them. But now the positive side is that I am getting to know them now'. Respondent 20. 'I am glad that I am getting more time with my children and husband'. Respondent 16.
		Persistent Gender inequalities	The persistence of the idea that men and women are not equal, and this would influence their experience of life.	'Household chores are mostly women's work. But my husband helps when I ask him to'. Respondent 2. 'My husband helps but not much. It's too much work for a single individual but that is the setback of the society'. Respondent 1.

Table 3.1 (Continued)

S. No.	*Theme*	*Subtheme*	*Descriptors*	*Examples*
3.	Impact on workload	The blurring of personal and professional boundaries	Diffusion of line between the personal and professional work hours	'Workload at home has increased because we have no domestic workers working right now. But overall activity has decreased. Lifestyle has become more sedentary. And now so much work is being done on video calls that it is affecting my time with family and children'. Respondent 12.
		Work-family conflict	Expansion of work and increase in domestic burden affect one another	'My kids now have to help me with PPT and technology. Everything has changed. So, though I know I must take their help as so much time has passed since I used computers'. Respondent 16. 'The increased workload is affecting my time as well as my time with the family'. Respondent 4.
		Reduced access to the informal network at work	Reduced opportunity for face-to-face networking	'I used to enjoy working and talking to my clients. After the lockdown that stopped and now my husband has not been permitted to go back to work. So, I see no opportunity for career growth'. Respondent 20.
		The blurring of gender roles	Reduction in adherence to rigid gender roles or expectations	'Husband and kids help. Cooking three times is difficult for anyone'. Respondent 16.

(*Continued*)

Table 3.1 (Continued)

S. No.	*Theme*	*Subtheme*	*Descriptors*	*Examples*
		Rise in domestic workload	Increase in domestic chores and responsibilities	'Although I am not working that much from home still work has increased at home. Now I am doing cooking and cleaning and do not have any domestic help that I had earlier'. Respondent 13.
4	Coping	Habituation	a decrease in response to a stimulus after repeated exposure	'Now we are past that panic stage. We have become used to the changes that are happening'. Respondent 4.
		Forced adjustment	the alterations made in behaviour to achieve the desired fit.	'It is difficult to manage work and home. But we have no other option but to do it'. Respondent 15.

Psychological and Emotional Health

COVID-19 and the associated social distancing norms were found to have psychological and emotional health consequences for married women. The participants reported experiencing several negative outcomes in the form of feelings of being immured, anxiety ambivalence, or mixed feelings.

Immured

Several participants reported feeling immured. It refers to the feelings of being trapped or caged. Several participants reported that they felt 'trapped' as they could not go out of their houses due to the lockdown. Moreover, these feelings were worsened by a desire to return to the state that existed before the pandemic. These feelings were expressed in several narratives such as:

> In the current situation, I feel trapped. Even in the beginning, we were caged. We were at home and could not go out.
>
> (Respondent 6)

> I feel bound and feel that my freedom has gone.
>
> (Respondent 20)

Anxiety

Anxiety refers to the negative feelings of apprehension. The participants reported feeling anxious about contracting the disease and due to other stressors associated with the pandemic. These include economic instability and conditions of uncertainty, among others. This anxiety was manifested in narratives such as:

> There was anxiety. My anxiety had increased. And there was no real social support. Everything was virtual. It was not a particularly good feeling.
>
> (Respondent 3)

Ambivalence/Mixed Feelings

Ambivalence refers to a state of conflicting feelings both partly positive and partly negative. Several participants reported having ambivalent feelings about the impact of the imposed lockdown. Such ambivalence can be discomforting for the individuals. Several narratives of the participants were found to reflect the discomfort resulting from the experience of ambivalence/mixed feelings. For instance:

> The experience of the lockdown was okay. I can say 50-50. I had mixed feelings. I liked something and disliked some things.
>
> (Respondent 15)

Social Impact

It is a well-established fact that social support is crucial for human beings. Being social beings, humans strive for connectedness with other humans (Corey, 2009). However, social distancing norms resulted in barriers to social interactions. Consequently, many people felt socially disconnected. On the other hand, being able to spend more time with immediate family members at home resulted in increased intimacy among them. Three subthemes emerged under social impact categorically namely 'social isolation, emotional intimacy and persistent gender inequalities' under the major theme of social impact.

Social Isolation

Social isolation refers to a state of complete or near-complete lack of contact between an individual and society. Several participants in the present study reported feeling disconnected and socially isolated. These feelings were reflected in narratives such as:

> Close relations continue but otherwise the pandemic has left an emotional impact. We cannot meet people and relatives we used to. I feel there is a disconnect.
>
> (Respondent 2)

Emotional Intimacy

Due to the hassles of daily life, people were often unable to spend quality time with their family. However, due to the imposed lockdowns, people were confined to their homes with their family as they worked from home. Consequently, several people were able to develop better emotional bonds with their family members. Several participants reported experiencing increased emotional intimacy in the form of improved emotional bonding with their immediate family members. This was reflected in several narratives such as:

> Now that I am spending more time at home, I am valuing more things, especially more time with family.
>
> (Respondent 1)

> I feel I am getting more time with my husband. The equation of working from home with your loved one is much better.
>
> (Respondent 6)

Persistent Gender Inequalities

Social impact could also be observed in the form of persistent gender inequalities. It refers to the persistence of the idea that men and women are not equal, and this would influence their experience of life. COVID-19 had a differential impact on men and women as existing gender inequalities were observed to be exacerbated in some cases. The narratives of various participants were indicative of these gender inequalities. For instance:

> My husband did not allow me to work from home during the lockdown and even now he is not allowing. I hope my in-laws will understand what it means for me and will allow me to go back to work.
>
> (Respondent 20)

Moreover, it was also observed that many women had accepted these inequalities as a norm and despite disproportionately sharing domestic responsibilities with their male counterparts did not report a need to receive more help. For instance, one participant reported:

> My husband and kids are helping me with household work. Whatever they are doing is sufficient. What if we do not even get this much help?
>
> (Respondent 9)

Impact on Workload

Another major theme that emerged in the narratives was related to the impact of the pandemic on workload. The COVID-19 pandemic witnessed a major transition in the professional world as people tried to adapt to the crisis situation. Several professions shifted to virtual platforms as people began working from homes. With people spending more time at home, males began noticing the number of domestic responsibilities that women were taking up. In some cases, domestic responsibilities further increased due to the non-availability and discontinuation of paid domestic help and more hours being spent at home. The impact on the workload for married women could be observed in the following areas.

The blurring of personal and professional boundaries, work–family conflicts, reduced access to informal networks at home resulted in rise in domestic workload. One positive impact could also be observed in the form of the blurring of gender role boundaries.

The Blurring of Personal and Professional Boundaries

The COVID-19 pandemic witnessed a diffusion of the fine line that existed between personal and professional life. Working from home resulted in the absence of a separate workspace for most of the people. Most professions started expecting individuals to stretch beyond the usual work hours some of which was lost due to internet-related issues. Also, many individuals found adapting to modern technology difficult and required more time to complete the professional tasks resulting in the encroachment of personal time by professional time. This could be observed in various narratives such as:

> Earlier there were boundaries. Now there is no fixed time to get up and go to sleep. You do not know when the day starts and when it ends.
>
> (Respondent 5)

> Boundaries have extended a lot. Earlier working till 7 pm was considered to be late. Now working even till 10:30 pm in the night is considered to be normal.
>
> (Respondent 6)

Work–Family Conflict

Work–family conflict refers to the reciprocal negative impact that the expansion of professional workload and increased domestic burden have mutually. Due to the blurring of professional and personal boundaries and sudden transitions in the work culture, several people witnessed a drastic increase in professional responsibilities and workload. Moreover, due to the fear of the spread of the disease, most families discontinued receiving support from paid domestic help. Also, the imposed lockdown and social distancing norms required people to avoid going out and spend more time at home. As a result, was an increase in the domestic workload in addition to the professional workload. Existing gender inequalities placed greater demands on women, particularly married women to strike a balance between work and family life thus creating a work–family conflict. This was reflected in several narratives of the participants such as:

> I used to worry about working from home. That during calls everyone else must remain quiet at my expense. And it gives me chills thinking about working from home during winters when fans and ACs cannot drown background noises.
>
> (Respondent 6)

Reduced Access to the Informal Network at Work

Informal social networks at the workplace often offer opportunities for personal growth and social support. However, in the work-from-home scenarios, the opportunities for informal networking decreased. Moreover, women were often able to devote less time to online professional activities in comparison to men because they shared a greater load of domestic responsibilities. Consequently, such a transition negatively impacted a married woman's career growth. For instance, one participant reported:

> I used to enjoy working and talking to my clients. After the lockdown that stopped and now my husband has not been permitted to go back to work. So, I see no opportunity for career growth.
>
> (Respondent 20)

Rise in Domestic Workload

Several participants reported an increase in the domestic workload and responsibilities that they shared disproportionately in comparison to their male counterparts. Various narratives were indicative of the rise in domestic workload due to the discontinuation of paid domestic help and a greater number of people spending more time at home. For instance:

> During lockdown work has increased. Cooking has increased because all the males are at home. My husband has no schedule. He gets up late, then I must make breakfast for him.
>
> (Respondent 20)

The Blurring of Gender Roles

Among various negative outcomes for married women, one positive outcome that could be observed was the blurring of gender roles. It refers to the reduction in adherence to rigid gender roles or expectations. As men began spending more time at home during the lockdown, the unpaid labour of women became more apparent to them. Consequently, some men even offered to help their wives and mothers in the domestic chores that were once considered to be feminine tasks. For instance, one participant reported:

> I have been receiving help in all the areas from my husband. Then my mother-in-law also helps.
>
> (Respondent 6)

Coping

For any individual sudden transitions in any sphere of life can be difficult and overwhelming. The conditions involving the COVID-19 pandemic and the imposed social distancing measures were no different. The personal and professional lives of the people were significantly changed in a short period influencing their physical and mental health. Hence, every individual tries to cope with such circumstances in his/her way. Two dominant coping styles, i.e., habituation and forced adjustment emerged from the narratives.

Habituation

Habituation can be defined as a decrease in response to a stimulus after repeated exposure. When COVID-19 began spreading at the beginning of the year 2020 and the social distancing norms had been recently imposed the anxiety, fear of contracting the disease, and feelings of uncertainty were more intense. However, as the time elapsed participants reported a reduction in these feelings as they got habituated to the existing conditions. For instance, one participant reported:

> This pandemic situation is challenging but it is going to persist for some time. So now I am getting used to the social distancing norms.
>
> (Respondent 19)

Some participants even reported that not only did such habituation helped them to cope with the circumstances but also enabled them to acquire healthy hygiene habits and routines that would be beneficial for them in the long run. For example, one participant shared:

> These social distancing norms have now become our habits. These are going to be helpful for everyone if they continue to persist later also.
>
> (Respondent 10)

Forced Adjustment

The adjustment refers to the alterations made in the behaviour to meet the desired fit. Though participants reported that the changes made in behavioural repertoires would have long-term benefits, many reported that these changes were not made willingly. The need for adjustment was forced upon them due to the contagious nature of the COVID-19 disease. For instance:

> Though adjustment to the COVID-19 pandemic is taking a toll on physical and mental health, we have no other option. We will have to adjust.
>
> (Respondent 2)

Discussion

The COVID-19 pandemic was not a sheer health issue. It was also an insightful shock to our societies and economies, with women being at the epicentre (United Nations Women, 2020). The easiest way to prevent the risk of infection from COVID-19, in the absence of any known vaccine, was, to embrace the practice of social distancing. Though the pandemic paradox had an impact on both males and females, the experience of it was different for the two genders. COVID-19 highlighted gender inequality in several areas ranging from domestic burden to economic outcomes. The present study was conducted on married women to explore their experiences during COVID-19 concerning the imposed social distancing norms. It further explored the possible role of social distancing measures in increasing gender inequality during COVID-19.

The findings of the present study are not only consistent with the findings of several other studies that have reported similar findings (Alon et al., 2020; McLaren et al., 2020; Levine, 2020; Lewin & Rasmussen, 2020;) but also highlight the emotional and psychological impact of COVID-19 on married women. Participants of the present study reported the significant impact on social life and workload and shared the coping strategies being practised by them during COVID-19.

The findings indicated that participants experienced several negative outcomes in the form of feelings of being immured, i.e., the participants felt 'trapped' as they could not go out of their homes due to mobility restrictions. Moreover, such feelings were worsened by the desire to return to the state that existed before the pandemic. Economic instability and conditions of uncertainty were stressors that were found to be associated with such feelings (Dwason et al., 2020; Miglani, 2020; Musinguzi et al., 2020). Ambivalence was also evidently reported in the study, involving expressions of mixed feelings about the impact of the imposed lockdown. Research indicates that uncertainty induces ambivalence, and such feelings can be discomforting (Fischer et al., 2020; Harreveld et al., 2009).

The present study further revealed that social distancing norms resulted in barriers to social interactions. Corey in 2009 found that social support is crucial for human beings. Being social beings, humans strive for connectedness with other humans. However, being able to spend more time with immediate family members at home resulted in increased intimacy among them. In exploring the impact on social life, social isolation, emotional intimacy, and persistent gender inequalities during COVID-19 emerged as dominant themes. Participants reported feelings of being disconnected and socially isolated during the pandemic.

In assessing the impact of workload in times of COVID-19, the study found a blurring of personal and professional boundaries. In other words, it refers to the diffusion of personal life and professional life. Working from home resulted in the absence of a separate workspace for most people (Bouziri et al., 2020; Ipsen et al, 2020; Bick et al., 2020; Kramer, 2020). During COVID-19, several organisations began expecting their employees to work beyond the usual work hours, to compensate for the loss in the same due to technological glitches. It was also difficult for some individuals to get acquainted with the technological skills required for the novel transitions resulting in encroachment of the personal time by the professional time (Merrifield, 2020; Baker et al., 2020; Nakroseine et al., 2019; Middleton, 2008).

The findings also indicated major transitions in the work culture due to the intermixing of personal and professional boundaries, along with a drastic increase in professional responsibilities and workload. Moreover, due to the fear of the spread of the disease, most families discontinued receiving support from paid domestic help, resulting in increase in workload which led to the work–life conflict. Due to the imposed lockdown and social distancing norms, married women, and other family members were spending more time at home. This resulted in an increment in the domestic workload in addition to the professional workload. Studies in the past have also reported that demands to strike a balance between work and family life were greater in women resulting in work–family conflict (Park et al., 2011; Shumate, 2004). Women as a whole, including those in formal sectors experienced increased burdens of caretaking for children, family members, and their homes with school closings, confinement, and lack of access to essential services during the pandemic (Asia and Pacific, United Nations Women, 2020).

Access to informal social networks at the workplace often offers opportunities for personal growth and social support. However, in the work-from-home scenarios, the opportunities for informal networking considerably decreased (Makison, 2012). Moreover, women were not able to devote much time to professional activities as compared to men because they shared a greater load of domestic responsibilities. Consequently, such a transition negatively impacted a married woman's career growth (Madgavkar et al., 2020; Noonan, 2020).

The close proximity among family members due to mobility restrictions made people to develop better emotional bonds with their family members. Another positive impact could also be observed in the form of distortion of gender role boundaries. Reichelt et al. (2020) also indicated that gender-role attitudes co-evolve and shape employment relationships and such bonding might be adapted to the realities of COVID-19.

Every individual tries to cope with COVID-19 related uncertain circumstances in his/her own way. In the present study, it was found that habituation and forced adjustment were the two dominant coping strategies practised by married women. The coping styles were different during the initial spread of the pandemic (Dwason, 2020; Wang, 2020). However, as the time elapsed participants reported a reduction in these feelings as they got habituated to the existing conditions. Costa et al. (2022) demonstrated that active coping strategies and increased social support were significantly correlated with decreased psychological distress. Moreover, the findings of our study also suggest that habituation was helpful for married women to cope with the crisis of COVID-19 and also facilitated the acquiring of healthy hygiene habits and routines that would be beneficial for them in the long run (Bin Abdulrahman et al., 2019).

This study also found that some changes that were made in the behavioural repertoires of married women might have long-term benefits, however, those changes were not willingly made by them. Henceforth, the need for adjustment was forced upon them due to the contagious nature of the COVID-19 disease. Such a negative style of coping may lead to hostility. Duan et al. (2020) also concluded that the use of negative coping strategies plays a potential intermediating role in the stress-related increase in hostility, while social support acts as a buffer in hostility in the general population under high stress. Kuang et al. (2020) found evidence revealing that fear and changes in stress levels may serve as a reference in suggesting coping strategies and designing programs with a focus on mental well-being based on the findings of our study.

These findings collectively demonstrate that married women were impacted not only emotionally but psychologically as well during the pandemic. They also experienced a significant detrimental impact on the support they used to get socially; their workload was also affected significantly. And lastly, they are continuously trying to cope with the pandemic and the associated social distancing norms by using coping styles such as habituation and forced adjustment.

Conclusion, Limitations, and Implications

The present research was conducted to develop an understanding of the experiences of married women during the COVID-19 pandemic and the period of imposed social distancing norms to understand the shift in gender roles, choices, and consequences. However, these experiences have not been compared with that of married or unmarried men. Based on some other published research, it could be observed that some of the experiences are shared by both men and women alike. However, the fact that women disproportionately shared the domestic workload and experienced persistent gender inequalities made their experience of the COVID-19 pandemic more adverse. Also, the current research did not explore the possibility and prevalence of gender-based violence and domestic violence with the participants at the time of the research and primarily focused on adherence to gender roles.

Compliance with Ethical Standards

The authors of this manuscript do not have any conflict of interest. The study was conducted in the absence of any funding and the informed consent from all participants was recorded before beginning the interviews. The study is conducted following APA's code of ethics for psychological research as well as according to the Helsinki Declaration.

References

Alon, T. M., Olmstead-Rumsey, J., Doepke, M., & Tertilt, M. (2020). The impact of COVID-19 on gender equality. *Working Paper*. Available online at www.nber.org/system/files/working_papers/w26947/w26947.pdf (accessed Oct 20, 2020).

Andrew, A., Cattan, S., Dias, M. C., Farquharson, C., Kraftman, L., Krutikova, S., ... & Sevilla, A. (2020). *How Are Mothers and Fathers Balancing Work and Family Under Lockdown?* United Kingdom: Institute for Fiscal Studies.

Baker, S. R., Bloom, N., Davis, S. J., & Terry, S. J. (2020). COVID-induced economic uncertainty (Working Paper No. 26983). National Bureau of Economic Research. www.nber.org/papers/w26983

Bick, A., Blandin, A., & Mertens, K. (2020). Work from home after the Covid-19 outbreak (Working Paper). Federal Bank of Dallas. Accessed at www.researchgate.net/publication/343038714_Work_from_Home_After_the_COVID-19_Outbreak/citations#fullTextFileContent

Bin Abdulrahman, A. K., Bin Abdulrahman, K. A., Almadi, M. K., Alharbi, A. M., Mahmoud, M. A., Almasri, M. S., Alanazi, T. R., Alarifi, R. A., Kilani, A. A., Albluwi, O. S., Al Fraih, M. A., Al Otabi, Y. T., Alanazi, H. O., Almufarih, W. A., Alokayli, A. M., & Alwhibi, O. A. (2019). Do various personal hygiene habits protect us against influenza-like illness? *BMC Public Health, 19*(1), 1324. https://doi.org/10.1186/s12889-019-7726-9.

Bouziri, H., Smith, D. R. M., Descatha, A., et al. (2020). Working from home in the time of COVID-19: how to best preserve occupational health? *Occupational and Environmental Medicine*, *77*, 509–510.

Braun, V. & Clarke, V. (2006). Using thematic analysis in psychology. *Qualitative Research in Psychology, 3*, 77–101.

Carlson, D. L., Petts, R., & Pepin, J. (2021). Changes in US parents' domestic labor during the early days of the COVID-19 pandemic. *Sociological Inquiry, 92*(3). https://doi.org/10.1111/soin.12459

Ciciolla, L., & Luthar, S. S. (2019). Invisible household labour and ramifications for adjustment: mothers as captains of households. *Sex Roles*, *81*(7–8), 467–486.

Collins, C., Landivar, L. C., Ruppanner, L., & Scarborough, W. J. (2021). COVID-19 and the gender gap in work hours. *Gender, Work, and Organisation*, *28*(Suppl 1), 101–112. https://doi.org/10.1111/gwao.12506

Corey, G. (2009). *Theories and Practices of Counseling and Psychotherapy*. Belmont, CA: Thomson Brooks/Cole.

Costa, M. A., Kristensen, C. H., Dreher, C. B., Manfro, G. G., & Salum, G.A. (2022). Habituating to pandemic anxiety: Temporal trends of COVID-19 anxiety over sixteen months of COVID-19. *Journal of Affective Disorders, 313*, 32–35. doi: 10.1016/j.jad.2022.06.077

Craig, L., & Brown, J. E. (2017). Feeling rushed: Gendered time quality, work hours, nonstandard work schedules, and spousal crossover. *Journal of Marriage and Family*, *79*(1), 225–242.

Craig, L., & Churchill, B. (2021). Dual-earner parent couples' work and care during COVID-19. *Gender, Work, and Organization*, *28*(Suppl 1), 66–79. https://doi.org/10.1111/gwao.12497.

Czymara, C. S., Langenkamp, A., & Cano, T. (2020). Cause for concern: Gender inequality in experiencing the COVID-19 lockdown in Germany. *European Societies*, 1–14.

Dawson, D. L., & Golijani-Moghaddam, N. (2020). COVID-19: Psychological flexibility, coping, mental health, and wellbeing in the UK during the pandemic. *Journal of Contextual Behavioral Science, 17*, 126–134. https://doi.org/10.1016/j.jcbs.2020.07.010

Duan, H., Yan, L., Ding, X., Gan, Y., Kohn, N., & Wu, J. (2020). Impact of the COVID-19 pandemic on mental health in the general Chinese population: Changes, predictors, and psychosocial correlates. *Psychiatry Research, 293*. https://doi.org/10.1016/j.psychres.2020.113396

Farré, L., Fawaz, Y., González, L., & Graves, J. (2021). Gender inequality in paid and unpaid work during Covid-19 times. *The Review of Income and Wealth, 68*(2). https://doi.org/10.1111/roiw.12563

Fischer, I., Avrashi, S., Oz T., Fadul R., Gutman K., Rubenstein D., Kroliczak G., Goerg S., & Glöckner A. (2020). The behavioural challenge of the COVID-19 pandemic: Indirect measurements and personalized attitude changing treatments (IMPACT). *Royal Society Open Science, 7*. https://doi.org/10.1098/rsos.201131

Harreveld, F. V., Rutjens, B., Nordgren, L. F., & Pligt, J. (2009). Ambivalence and decisional conflict as a cause of psychological discomfort: Feeling tense before jumping off the fence. *Journal of Experimental Social Psychology, 54*, 167–173. https://doi.org/10.1016/j.jesp.2008.08.015

Hennekam, S., & Shymko, Y. (2020). Coping with the COVID-19 crisis: *Force majeure* and gender performativity. *Gender, Work, and Organization, 27*(5), 788–803. https://doi.org/10.1111/gwao.12479

Hjálmsdóttir, A., & Bjarnadóttir, V. S. (2021). "I have turned into a foreman here at home": Families and work–life balance in times of COVID-19 in a gender equality paradise. *Gender, Work and Organization, 28*(1), 268–283. https://doi.org/10.1111/gwao.12552

Hodgkinson, T., & Andresen, M. A. (2020). Show me a man or a woman alone and I will show you a saint: changes in the frequency of criminal incidents during the COVID-19 pandemic. *Journal of Criminal Justice, 69*, 101706.

Hussain, H., Hussain, S., Zahra, S., & Hussain, T. (2020). Prevalence and risk factors of domestic violence and its impacts on women's mental health in Gilgit-Baltistan, Pakistan. *Pakistan Journal of Medical Sciences, 36*(4), 627–631.

International Labour Organisation. [ILO] (2020). "*ILO Monitor: COVID-19 and the World of Work, Third Edition*", Geneva, available at: www.ilo.org/wcmsp5/groups/public/@dgreports/@dcomm/documents/briefing note/wcms_743146.pdf (Accessed: Oct 28, 2020).

Ipsen, C., & Kirchner, K., & Hansen, J. (2020). Experiences of working from home in times of COVID-19. *An International Survey Conducted the First Months of the National Lockdowns.* https://doi.org/10.11581/dtu:00000085

Kramer, A., & Kramer, K. Z. (2020). The potential impact of the COVID-19 pandemic on occupational status, work from home, and occupational mobility. *Journal of Vocational Behavior, 119*, 103442. https://doi.org/10.1016/j.jvb.2020.103442

Kuang, J., Ashraf, S., Das, U., & Bicchieri, C. (2020). Awareness, risk perception, and stress during the COVID-19 pandemic in communities of Tamil Nadu, India. *International Journal of Environmental Research and Public Health, 17*, 7177.

Lee, E., & Frayn, E. (2008). The 'feminisation' of health. In *A Sociology of Health* (pp. 115–133). SAGE Publications Ltd. https://doi.org/10.4135/9781446213575

Levine, S. (2020). Paradox of quarantine: humans are coming together. *Psychology Today.* Available online at: www.psychologytoday.com/intl/blog/our-emotional-footprint/202004/the-paradox-quarantine-humans-are-coming-together (accessed Oct 28, 2020).

Madgavkar, A., White O., Krishnan M., Mahajan, D., & Azcue, X. (2020). *COVID-19 and Gender Equality: Countering the Regressive Effects*. New York: McKinsey Global Institute. Available online at: www.mckinsey.com/featured-insights/future-of-work/covid-19-and-gender-equality-countering-the-regressive-effects (accessed: Oct 24, 2020).

Maji, S., Bansod, S., & Singh, T. (2022). Domestic violence during COVID-19 pandemic: The case for Indian women. *Journal of Community & Applied Social Psychology, 32*(3), 374–381. https://doi.org/10.1002/casp.2501

Manzo, L. K. C., & Minello, A. (2020). Mothers, childcare duties, and remote working under COVID-19 lockdown in Italy: Cultivating communities of care. *Dialogues in Human Geography*, 2043820620934268.

McLaren, H. J., Wong, K. R., Nguyen, k. N., & Mahamadachchi, K. N. D. (2020). COVID-19 and women's triple burden: Vignettes from Sri Lanka, Malaysia, Vietnam, and Australia. *Social Sciences,* 9, 87.

Merrifield, C. (2020) *Working from Home: What the Research Says about Setting Boundaries, Staying Productive and Reshaping Cities*. Harvard Kennedy School, Shorenstein Center on Media, Politics and Public Policy. Available online at https://journalistsresource.org/studies/economics/jobs/working-from-home-telework-research/ (accessed Oct 24, 2020).

Middleton, C. A. (2008). Do mobile technologies enable work-life balance? In Hislop, D. (ed.), *Mobility and Technology in the workplace* (pp. 209–224). Abingdon: Routledge.

Miglani, A. (2020). Effect of lockdown during COVID-19: An Indian perspective. *International Journal of Science & Healthcare Research, 5*(3), 55–61.

Mittal, S., & Singh, T. (2020). Gender-based violence during COVID-19 pandemic: A mini-review. *Frontiers in Global Womens Health, 1*, 4.

Musinguzi, G., & Asamoah, B. O. (2020). The COVID-19 lockdown trap, how do we get out? *Journal of Clinical and Experimental Investigations, 11*(4), https://doi.org/10.29333/jcei/8343

Nakrošienė, A., Bučiūnienė, I., & Goštautaitė, B. (2019). Working from home: Characteristics and outcomes of telework. *International Journal of Manpower, 40*(1), 87–101. https://doi.org/10.1108/IJM-07-2017-0172

Noonan, M. (2001). The impact of domestic work on men's and women's wages. *Journal of Marriage and Family, 63*(4), 1134–1145. https://doi.org/10.1111/j.1741-3737.2001.01134.x

Park, Y., Fritz, C., & Jex, S.M. (2011) Relationships between work-home segmentation and psychological detachment from work: The role of communication technology use at home. *Journal of Occupational Health Psychology, 16*(4), 457–467.

Qian, Y., & Fuller, S. (2020). COVID-19 and the gender employment gap among parents of young children. *Canadian Public Policy, 46*(S2), S89–S101.

Reichelt, M., Makovi, K., & Sargsyan, A. (2020). The impact of COVID-19 on gender inequality in the labour market and gender-role attitudes. *European Societies*, https://doi.org/10.1080/14616696.2020.1823010

Robertson, L. G., Anderson, T. L., Hall, M. E. L., & Kim, C. L. (2019). Mothers and mental labor: A phenomenological focus group study of family-related thinking work. *Psychology of Women Quarterly, 43*(2), 184–200.

Shumate, M., & Fulk, J. (2004) Boundaries and role conflict: When work and family are co-located: a communication network and symbolic interaction approach. *Human Relations, 57*, 55–74.

Uchoa, P. (2020). Coronavirus: Will women have to work harder after the pandemic? *BBC World Service.* Available online at www.bbc.com/news/business-53363253 (accessed Oct 24, 2020).

United Nations Women Asia and the Pacific [UN Women] (2020). *The Impact of COVID-19 on Women's Burden of Care and Unpaid Domestic Labor.* Available online at: https://asiapacific.unwomen.org/en/digital-library/publications/2020/05/the-impact-of-covid-19-on-womens-burden-of-care-and-unpaid-domestic-labor (accessed Oct 23, 2020).

United Nations Women [UN Women] (2020). *In Focus: Gender Equality Matters in COVID-19 Response.* Available online at www.unwomen.org/en/news/in-focus/in-focus-gender-equality-in-covid-19-respone, (accessed Oct 21, 2020).

Wang H, Xia Q, Xiong Z, Li Z, Xiang W, Yuan Y, et al. (2020) The psychological distress and coping styles in the early stages of the 2019 coronavirus disease (COVID-19) epidemic in the general mainland Chinese population: A web-based survey. *PLoS ONE, 15*(5). https://doi.org/10.1371/journal.pone.0233410

Wenham, C., Smith, J., & Morgan, R. (2020). Gender and COVID-19 Working Group. COVID-19: The gendered impacts of the outbreak. *Lancet, 395*(10227), 846–848.

Yu, H., Li, M., Li, Z., et al. (2020). Coping style, social support, and psychological distress in the general Chinese population in the early stages of the COVID-19 epidemic. *BMC Psychiatry, 20*, 426. https://doi.org/10.1186/s12888-020-02826-3

4 Resilience Amidst Adversity

Exploration of Undergraduate Students Post-COVID-19 Experiences in Kerala

Soumya T Varghese and Vineetha K J

Introduction

Kerala, a southern state in India, encountered the COVID-19 pandemic with both resilience and challenges. As of the latest data mentioned in the Government of Kerala State Dashboard (Go KDasboard) dated September 2022, Kerala has reported 6,767,856 confirmed cases, with a recovery rate of 98.8%. However, the state also faced 70,913 deaths (mortality rate—1.047%), highlighting the severity of the virus's impact. The test positivity rate has been closely monitored, standing at 2.04% on average. The state's resilience lies not only in its numbers but also in the strong support systems provided by educational institutions, families, and peers (Vinod & Kini, 2022). Resilience is defined as the culmination of self-awareness, determination, vision, self-confidence, organisation, problem-solving, interaction, and relationships (Mowbray, 2014). Resilience was fostered by the support systems provided by communities and educational institutions. As a result of varied collaborative efforts, there were multiple coping strategies to address various challenges. Together, Kerala quite successfully navigated the uncertainties of the pandemic, emphasising the importance of community connections and determination in overcoming adversity (Ali & George, 2021). The COVID-19 pandemic has had a profound impact on the lives of many and among them, the student population were the most affected and their mental health concerns have gained increasing attention among researchers (Salimi, 2023; Rafi et al., 2020). Mental health and wellbeing concerns were crucial for the student population as the epidemic created new stressors for them, leaving an indelible mark on their perspectives towards resilience. The marked lifestyle changes brought about by the COVID-19 pandemic, such as isolation, quarantine, and a complete shift to digital learning, have created a chaotic scenario that demanded considerable psycho-social effort to settle down. For many undergraduate students, accustomed to the rhythms of campus life and face-to-face interactions, the sudden transition to remote learning and social isolation has been disorienting (Morato et al., 2023). Gone were the days of bustling lecture halls and spontaneous gatherings with friends; instead, students find themselves navigating within the virtual classrooms and communicating through screens. For many students, the abrupt shift to online learning disrupted established

DOI: 10.4324/9781003517313-5

routines and social connections. The lack of in-person interactions, campus events, and extracurricular activities led to feelings of isolation and disconnection (Madhavan et al., 2022). The uncertainty surrounding the pandemic has only added to the upheaval, with fears about health, finances, and the future weighing heavily on young minds. Adapting to this new way of life requires resilience and perseverance, as students must not only adjust to the technical challenges of online learning but also find ways to cope with feelings of loneliness and isolation. Despite the chaos, however, many students have demonstrated remarkable resilience, finding comfort in virtual communities, cultivating new hobbies, and discovering innovative ways to connect with peers and professors (Fayez et al., 2023). These virtual connections brought meaning to social media platforms and started contributing to the quality of life. As they continue to navigate these turbulent times, the lessons learned and the strength gained undoubtedly shape their futures in profound ways (Madhavan et al., 2022).

The pandemic has highlighted existing inequalities, with marginalised students disproportionately affected by issues such as lack of access to technology or stable internet connections (Pattnaik et al., 2023). The lack of technology access and reliable internet connections has hindered their ability to participate in remote learning. Many students had active high-speed internet connections while some faced problems due to various reasons such as financial constraints, accessibility, dearth of service providers, and poor supplementary digital infrastructure (Rahman, 2021). This divide tends to exacerbate existing inequalities. Marginalised students faced greater disruptions due to school closures, limited resources, and the shift to online education. Additionally, the digital divide became more pronounced, as students from marginalised backgrounds faced challenges related to technology access and stable internet connections. Rafi et al. (2020) in their research article have quoted network connectivity, power failure, and availability of gadgets or familiarity with the digital platforms as areas of improvisation for students in Kerala. The impact of the pandemic on education has been profound, touching every facet of the system from admissions to common entrance examinations and projects. Stressors were omnipresent, necessitating resilience as an indispensable coping mechanism (Ang et al., 2022). Kerala stands as a poignant example, being the first state in the country to confront the pandemic and experience its severity first-hand (GoK Dashboard, 2022). Through these challenges, the resilience of educators, students, and administrators has been put to the test, highlighting the importance of adaptability and determination in navigating such unprecedented times. Despite these challenges, students have shown remarkable resilience, adapting to new modes of learning and finding innovative ways to stay connected with peers and mentors. As the world navigates towards recovery, the long-term impacts of pandemic on undergraduate students remain to be fully understood, but one thing is clear: the pandemic has reshaped their academic journeys and personal growth.

Amidst the distress caused by the pandemic, students have emerged as bold and resilient advocates of their academic progress. Their ability to adapt, innovate, and connect has been nothing short of inspiring. As lecture halls transformed into virtual spaces, students embraced digital platforms with determination. They were successfully navigated through asynchronous classes, video conferences, and online assessments, all while maintaining a sense of community and shared goals. Virtual coffee chats, study sessions, and collaborative projects bridged the physical gaps, reinforcing the importance of human connection. The concept of resilience was shaped through their personal experiences and helped them to prevent adverse events, tolerate challenges, and manage troubles. Mowbray (2014) defined resilience as an approach to strengthening wellbeing and performance through psychological processes like self-awareness, determination, vision, self-confidence, organisation, problem-solving, interaction, and relationships. The definition provided by Mowbray was used as the operational definition for resilience. The post-pandemic period helped the students to engage with their reflections. As they reflected on their inner strength the psychological process that contributes to resilience was also manifolded. The theoretical perspective of personal resilience (Mowbray, 2014) provides clarity and explains the personal reflections and the underlying psychological processes involved.

Research Objectives

The research objectives can be listed as measuring the resilience levels of undergraduate students' experiences, examining the dimensions of resilience, and addressing the role of socio-demographic factors to understand the specific challenges and adversities faced by undergraduate students in Kerala in the post-pandemic period.

Hypotheses

Based on the objectives, the hypotheses can be listed as follows:

- The resilience levels of undergraduate students will exhibit significant variation among them.
- The resilience score will exhibit a significant correlation with the dimensions embedded such as self-awareness, determination, vision, self-confidence, organisation, problem-solving, interaction, and relationships.
- The resilience level of participants will exhibit significant differences concerning their age, geographical location, and chosen academic disciplines.

Method

Research Design

This research adopted a cross-cultural quantitative survey design to collect data from a sample of undergraduate students in Kerala (Rea & Parker, 2014). Students have participated from seven out of the total 14 districts of Kerala State.

Sample

A total of 85 participants (18 years and above) were drawn from various academic institutions and streams through a purposive sampling technique. The streams include Bachelor of Arts, Bachelor of Business Administration, Bachelor of Science, and Bachelor of Commerce. Informed written consent was obtained and participants were briefed about the study in detail.

Inclusion Criteria

Undergraduate students from Kerala who witnessed the COVID-19 pandemic during their graduation period. The inclusion criteria were based on geographical and temporal contexts. Geographically, the undergraduate students need to be from Kerala, and temporally, they had to be exposed to the COVID-19 pandemic during their graduation period.

Exclusion Criteria

Undergraduate students from regions other than Kerala who did not directly experience the COVID-19 pandemic during their graduation period.

Tools

The Resilience Assessment Questionnaire (RAQ) developed by Mowbray (2014) was used to measure resilience. It has two versions, the short form known as RAQ8, consists of eight questions, while the full version, RAQ40 contains 40 questions. It is a validated and widely used resilience assessment tool. The reliability of RAQ has not been tested as Mowbray claims that resilience is a generic attribute and not a situational one. As it is a contextually driven characteristic, being resilient in one situation may not provide any assurance of behaving in the same fashion the next time. In the RAQ, scores can range from 8 to 40. It is a Likert scale with five different options, where 1 shows 'never' and 5 shows 'always'. The scores for each category are summed and then combined to provide an overall resilience score. A score below 3 suggests a significant need to boost one's resilience (Mowbray, 2014; Horgan, 2014).

Data Collection

The data were collected online. The socio-demographic details and RAQ were consolidated into a single Google Form, which was then shared with student groups through various online platforms.

Data Analysis

The collected data were analysed with a Jamovi and non-parametric tests were used as data were not normally distributed. Descriptive statistics was employed to summarise and describe the general tendency of resilience. Spearman's correlational coefficient was calculated to examine the relationships among the components of resilience. Finally, Mann–Whitney *U* tests were conducted to identify significant differences in resilience scores based on discipline, location, and age.

Ethical Considerations

The Helsinki Guidelines were adhered to. The confidentiality of data was maintained.

Results of Categorisation of Resilience

The resilience levels of the participants have been investigated and classified into three distinct groups according to the high, low, and average scores. The categorisation of groups was done based on the mean score for resilience of 25.5 (SD = 5). The descriptive analysis reveals that 54% of the students fall within the average group, with 24% scoring in the higher range and 22% in the lower range. This distribution highlights the varying degrees of resilience among the students, with a significant proportion demonstrating an average level of resilience, while smaller percentages exhibit higher or lower levels (Figure 4.1).

Discussion

Resilience is an enduring inner strength which can act as a cornerstone in the holistic understanding of mental wellbeing (Rutter, 2023). The perspective reflects the idea that resilience is a choice, not a trait as mentioned by Mowbray (2014). It's a multifaceted construct, with both intrinsic and extrinsic characteristics. The

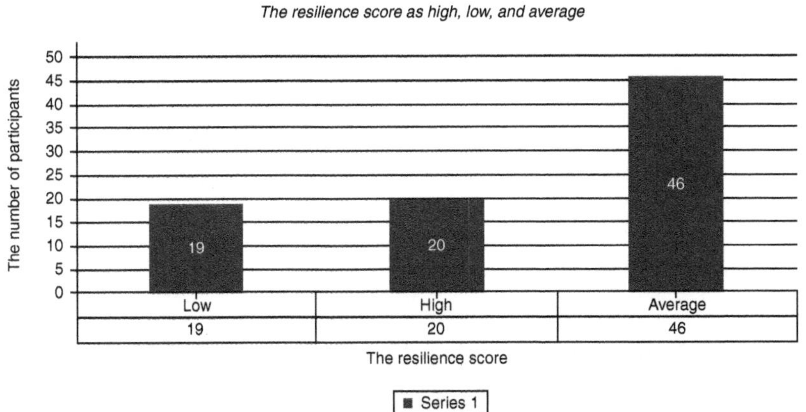

Figure 4.1 The resilience scores of the participants.

greater number of the participants fall within the average category. This trend may be due to the prevailing notion that resilience bears a robust link to life's tumultuous events and assumes a proactive role in such circumstances (Salzman, 2021). It's plausible that participants viewed their current situations through a lens of introspection during this research engagement. Resilience is a complex term that involves adaptability, optimism, and emotional regulation (Kireeva, 2022). These facets interlock, forming a resilient core for people to act upon. Researchers have taken resilience as a construct, examining its core structures which strengthen or contribute to the capacity to bounce back. Some of those factors are like amount of distress, vulnerability, and affect regulation as suggested by Grygorenko and Naydonova (2023). Identifiers—like the frequency of setbacks or the way we react—can be the basic building block for the struggle to be resilient.

The analysis of the percentages reveals that an equal half of the participants fell within the average category, both believing in and expressing resilience. This underscores the widespread recognition and importance placed on resilience as a vital component of psychological strength and coping mechanisms among students. However, there is a 22% discrepancy observed in the lower region of resilience. These variations may stem from differences in both intra and interpersonal factors (Sojer et al., 2024). Cassidy (2016) suggests that resilience is not a uniform trait across the broader population, but rather a multidimensional construct with psychological complexities. He further argues that resilience can defy expectations and can be viewed as an asset that can be cultivated into academic resilience, particularly within the context of education. This academic resilience serves as a valuable support during challenging times and can significantly enhance academic success. Building resilience, however, requires substantial resources, including adaptive, affective, and cognitive skills. This underscores the importance of investing in the development of these skills to bolster resilience and foster academic achievement, particularly in the face of adversity. The same fact can act as an explanatory mechanism for the deviations in the score into low, high, and average. The student community are in a position to adjust and adapt to the pandemic challenges and technology is getting more integrated into their existence (Comin et al., 2022). Currently, the turmoil they once experienced has merged itself into their collective identity. They now navigate significant life changes with ease, whether it involves learning or socialising on various platforms. Resilience is not a solitary intraindividual experience, but a collective community experience (Linnell, 2014). The emotional support they received from family, friends, mentors, and teachers to reassure, accept, and get engaged with their academic challenges helped them to navigate easily and adapt to the changes they were exposed to. Connectedness become a necessity for the student community and technology helped them to make it a reality.

Results of Correlation among the Embedded Dimensions of Resilience

The resilience score exhibited a significant correlation with the embedded dimensions.

Table 4.1 shows that vision and self-confidence exhibit high correlation (0.64). The problem-solving and determination have moderate correlations of 0.55 and

Table 4.1 The correlation among the dimensions of resilience

Correlation matrix										
		SA	*D*	*V*	*SC*	*O*	*PS*	*I*	*Rel*	*R*
Self-awareness (SA)	Spearman's rho	—								
	p-value	—								
Determination (D)	Spearman's rho	0.132	—							
	p-value	0.230	—							
Vision (V)	Spearman's rho	0.308 **	0.365 ***	—						
	p-value	0.004	<0.001	—						
Self-confidence (SC)	Spearman's rho	0.222 *	0.228 *	0.379 ***	—					
	p-value	0.041	0.036	<0.001	—					
Organisation (O)	Spearman's rho	0.258 *	0.170	0.114	0.190	—				
	p-value	0.017	0.120	0.299	0.082	—				
Problem-solving (PS)	Spearman's rho	0.095	0.192	0.168	0.371 ***	0.066	—			
	p-value	0.385	0.078	0.124	<0.001	0.548	—			
Interaction (I)	Spearman's rho	0.099	-0.013	0.052	0.205	-0.205	0.252 *	—		
	p-value	0.369	0.905	0.636	0.059	0.060	0.020	—		

(*Continued*)

Table 4.1 (Continued)

Correlation matrix																		
		SA		*D*		*V*		*SC*		*O*		*PS*		*I*		*Rel*		*R*
Relationship (Rel)	Spearman's rho	0.083		0.353	***	0.388	***	0.071		-0.001		0.282	**	0.306	**	—		
	p-value	0.448		<0.001		<0.001		0.520		0.994		0.009		0.004		—		
Resilience (R)	Spearman's rho	0.440	***	0.542	***	0.641	***	0.644	***	0.370	***	0.558	***	0.417	***	0.522	***	—
	p-value	<0.001		<0.001		<0.001		<0.001		<0.001		<0.001		<0.001		<0.001		—

Note. * $p < 0.05$, ** $p < 0.01$, *** $p < 0.001$

0.54, respectively. The dimension of relationship demonstrates a correlation of 0.52, while self-awareness follows with 0.44. Interaction and organisation show slightly lower correlations, with values of 0.41 and 0.37, respectively. These correlation values provide insights into the interplay between different dimensions of resilience and the overall resilience score, highlighting the significance of various factors in contributing to an individual's overall resilience level. Vision and self-confidence emerge as pivotal dimensions with above-average correlations (0.64) to resilience.

Discussion

Understanding oneself and acknowledging vulnerabilities are crucial aspects of fostering resilience. The ability to envision challenges and devise strategies to overcome them further enhances resilience. A closer examination of these components reveals their interconnected nature, indicating that the mechanisms underlying vision and self-confidence are intertwined. This insight underscores the importance of nurturing both aspects to cultivate a robust sense of resilience in individuals. That can happen through engagement, where one has to connect vision and self-confidence by being engaged with what they are pursuing (Cross, 2021). Following closely behind the vision and self-confidence, problem-solving, and determination emerge as significant dimensions of resilience. As individuals engage with their environments, they become exposed to increasingly challenging situations. Determination helps them to navigate through these obstacles, employing tactful problem-solving skills to overcome adversity. This active engagement and persistence in the face of challenges are integral to developing resilience, highlighting the importance of refining problem-solving abilities and fostering a determined mindset. Active engagement facilitated connections among students (Rutter, 2023). Virtual study groups, collaborative projects, and online discussions allowed students to share experiences, strategies, and emotional support. These interactions transcended disciplinary boundaries, creating a sense of community even in the digital realm. Engaged students maintained a sense of purpose. Regular participation in class discussions, attending virtual office hours, and actively contributing to coursework kept them motivated. The accountability of being part of a learning community encouraged consistent effort, even amidst the uncertainties of the pandemic. Active learners were quick to adapt. They explored new tools, sought out resources, and creatively addressed challenges. Whether troubleshooting technical issues or collaborating on group projects, their proactive approach bolstered their resilience (Prager, 2012). Engaging with peers and instructors provided a sense of normalcy and reduced feelings of isolation. Students who actively participated in online activities reported better emotional wellbeing. These connections served as a buffer against pandemic-related stressors.

Relationships and self-awareness emerge as the next dimensions with high scores, and interestingly, they are interconnected. Relationships that are founded on self-awareness—understanding oneself and how one connects with others—are particularly relevant. Understanding their learning preferences and strengths, students adapted their study routines. Some discovered that they thrived in quiet environments, while others found collaborative virtual spaces more conducive. Self-awareness enabled them to tailor their approach to online learning, optimising their productivity (Linnell, 2014). Self-aware students acknowledged their limitations. Whether related to time management, technology skills, or mental health, they sought support when needed. This awareness prevented burnout and allowed them to seek timely assistance from professors, counsellors, or peers. Reflecting on their values, goals, and aspirations, students reaffirmed their sense of purpose (Kireeva, 2022). Self-awareness prompted questions like What matters most to me? How can I contribute during this crisis? These reflections fuelled resilience by grounding students in their narratives.

Addressing a pandemic like COVID-19 was not a solitary endeavour; rather, it was a collective effort where individuals came together, adhered to regulations, and supported one another to overcome challenges (Prager, 2012). Relationships flourished through the cultivation of awareness, contributing significantly to resilience. This symbiotic relationship between self-awareness and relationships underscores their importance in navigating crises and building resilience collectively.

Interaction and organisation emerge as the final dimensions correlated with resilience, yet they remain crucial, particularly in the context of academic resilience. Amidst periods of complete isolation and detachment, how individuals interact with others and their ability to foster meaningful connections can significantly bolster resilience. Furthermore, organisational skills play a vital role; the capacity to identify and arrange resources in a controlled and structured manner supports resilience. A controlled and tranquil mindset is essential for effective organisation, allowing individuals to bring coherence to their surroundings. Effective organisational skills empower students to manage their academic responsibilities efficiently. When coursework shifted online, students had to juggle multiple tasks—attending virtual classes, submitting assignments, and studying independently (Grygorenko & Naydonova, 2023). The ability to prioritise, create schedules, and allocate time for each task became paramount. Organised students could break down complex assignments into smaller, manageable steps, reducing overwhelm. Moreover, maintaining a structured study environment—whether at home or in a shared space—enhanced focus and productivity. By arranging resources, setting reminders, and maintaining clear communication with professors, students fostered a sense of control over their academic lives. These organisational habits not only facilitated academic success but also bolstered their resilience. When faced with unexpected disruptions, students who had honed their organisational skills were better equipped to adapt swiftly and maintain a sense of stability.

Although the last in correlation, these components are instrumental in cultivating resilience, particularly in the academic realm, where effective interaction and organisation are indispensable for navigating challenges.

The resilience score of participants exhibited significant differences in their age, geographical location, and chosen disciplines.

Results on Comparison of Resilience Concerning Age

As per the Mann–Whitney *U* test, the age categories' differences are insignificant ($p = 0.849$).

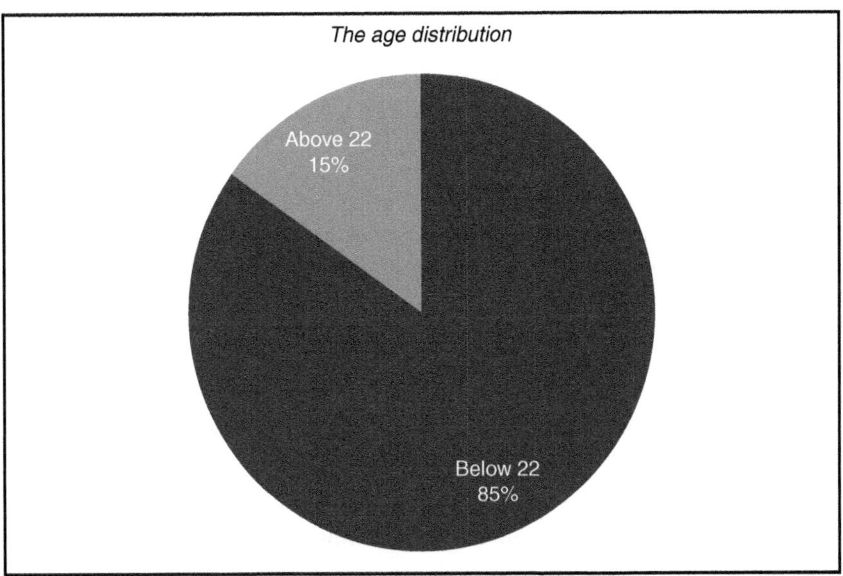

Figure 4.2 The age distribution of the participants.

Table 4.2 Resilience based on age

Mann–Whitney U test based on age			
		Statistic	*p*
Resilience	Mann–Whitney *U*	452	0.849

Note. $H_a\ \mu_1 \neq \mu_2$

Discussion

The age factor did not show any discernible differences in resilience scores among the participants. This observation can likely be attributed to the uniform nature of the sample, consisting solely of undergraduate students. Given that all participants were at a similar stage in their academic journeys, age variations may not have exerted a significant influence on resilience levels. This uniformity within the sample group underscores the importance of considering contextual factors when interpreting research findings and highlights the need for further exploration into the determinants of resilience among specific demographic groups. When children receive support and warmth during their formative years, these nurturing roots become the foundation for their resilience in later life, allowing them to bounce back through adverse scenarios (Sun & Stewart, 2007). Students of all ages embraced adaptability. They shifted seamlessly between in-person and remote learning, adjusted to changing schedules, and redefined success. Older students, who had experienced previous crises, provided reassurance that resilience was possible. Younger students, who never had any exposure to such situations, embraced new ways of thinking. Resilience may not correlate with age due to its complex dimensionality. Research on wellbeing and resilience in relation to age has shown that age may not statistically correlate with resilience and wellbeing (Svence et al., 2015). Age cannot be understood as a single factor in the context of resilience, rather the all sorts developments associated with age in terms of human evolvement is connected to resilience. Social relations act as a protective factor for resilience as people grow older and can promote resilience in various social scenarios. Fuller-Iglesias, Sellars, and Antonucci (2008) discussed the role of age with respect to social relations as a facilitating factor for resilience. Together, they dismantled age-related stereotypes and embraced a shared commitment to overcoming adversity. Age-diverse student groups advocated for common causes. Whether advocating for mental health resources, equitable access to technology, or inclusive policies, their collective voices amplified resilience.

Results on Comparison of Resilience Concerning Geographical Location

As per the Mann–Whitney *U* test, the geographical location differences are insignificant ($p = 0.482$).

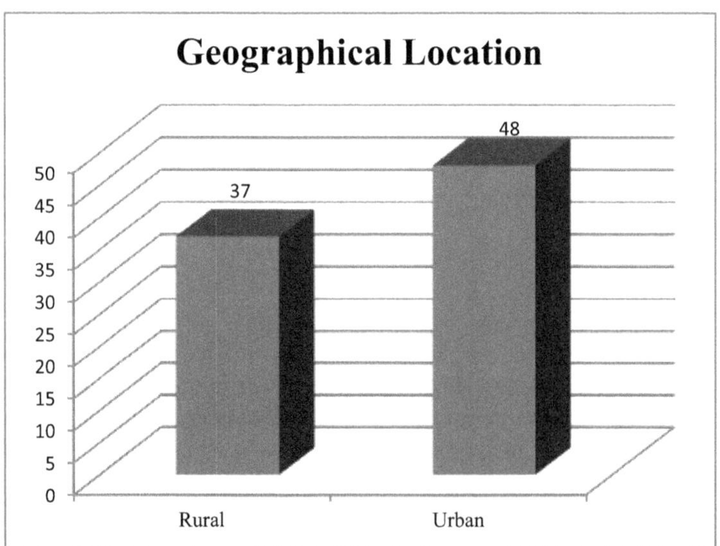

Figure 4.3 The distribution of geographical location.

Table 4.3 Resilience based on geographical location

Mann–Whitney U test			
		Statistic	*p*
Resilience	Mann–Whitney *U*	809	0.482

Note. H_a $\mu_1 \neq \mu_2$

Discussion

The geographical locations; urban and rural categories do not appear to have any discernible impact on the resilience. Despite variations in geographical borders within the state, students across different areas likely had access to information regarding the COVID-19 pandemic through various channels. This has been supported by the results depicted in Table 4.3. The dissemination of information appeared to occur uniformly, ensuring that students, regardless of their location, were exposed to similar challenges and circumstances. This uniformity suggests that external factors such as geographical location did not significantly influence the resilience levels observed among the student population, underscoring the widespread and consistent nature of the challenges posed by the pandemic as shown in Figure 4.3. Kerala state has received global acclaim for its swift response in containing the pandemic, despite being the first region to report a case. The state demonstrated remarkable resilience during the crisis, with students at the forefront, acting as dedicated COVID-warriors (Sundararaman et al, 2021). The collective efforts of Kerala's citizens exemplify the power of community resilience in overcoming adversity and will have a persistent influence on the student community. During the pandemic lockdown, a significant number of people returned to their homes, bridging the gap between urban and rural spaces. Rather than the vast outer world, individuals found solace in the familiar confines of their own homes. The usual spatial divide lost its relevance, and students, too, shared this unique pandemic experience. The shift in space transcended the geographical divide and the student community looked for familiar connections and interactions more through the digital space to manage the transition phase. The post-COVID-19 experiences are still happening on the same line as digital space helped students to access spaces which were not easily available before and helped them to redefine the concept of space. The pandemic-induced shift toward home spaces has profound implications for student development. Resilience perspectives in urban and rural areas are differentiated in terms of economic capital by Cutter, Ash, and Emrich (2016). They argue that economic capital acts as a strong driving factor for urban areas, whereas community capital is more significant for rural areas. As the urban–rural divide blurred, barriers related to physical space diminished opening up new spaces of possibilities. The once rigid boundaries between urban and rural become softened, allowing for a more meaningful exchange of ideas, experiences, and knowledge. No longer confined by geographical constraints, individuals found themselves interconnected in ways previously unimaginable. This transformation wasn't merely about traversing physical landscapes; it was a psychological shift through the realisation that shared humanity transcends borders and boundaries. Students, too, benefited from this expanded concept of digital space, accessing a global network of learning and collaboration (Mashayekhi & Mohammadi, 2014).

Results on Comparison of Resilience Concerning the Academic Discipline

As per the Kruskal–Wallis test, the disciplines' differences are insignificant ($\chi^2 = 4.35$).

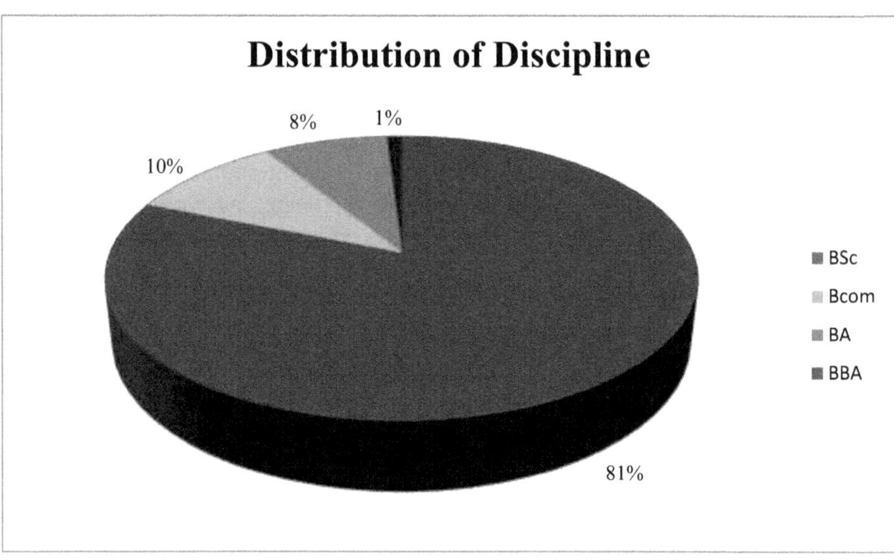

Figure 4.4 The distribution of discipline.

Table 4.4 Resilience based on the disciplines

Kruskal–Wallis				
	χ^2	*df*	*p*	ε^2
Resilience	4.35	3	0.226	0.0518

Discussion

The disciplines of the students did not seem to contribute to differences in resilience levels. It appears that regardless of their academic field, students similarly perceived challenges, suggesting a commonality in the experiences they faced. Issues such as accessing course content, submitting coursework, and interacting with professors were shared concerns among all students, irrespective of their specific discipline. This shared set of challenges likely played a significant role in minimising any differences in resilience based on discipline. The non-significant role of discipline in resilience could therefore be attributed to the uniformity of challenges encountered across all fields of study, highlighting the collective nature of the obstacles posed by the pandemic on undergraduate education. Under stressful situations, resilience can induce mindfulness and acts as a core component in a mindfulness program designed for undergraduate students. During the research, the experimental group demonstrated increased efficiency with resilience compared to the control group (Roulston et al., 2018).

The pandemic-induced disruptions to higher education transcended disciplinary boundaries, affecting students across all fields equally. The sudden shift to remote learning merged with technological glitches and limited access to resources, created a shared struggle for every student. Whether majoring in humanities, sciences, or engineering, the challenges were remarkably consistent: adapting to virtual classrooms, grappling with time zone differences, and navigating online platforms. As a result, the collective experience fostered a sense of solidarity among students, emphasising their shared resilience. The absence of significant discipline-based differences in resilience levels underscores the universality of these obstacles and the remarkable capacity of students to adapt collectively (Neville et al., 2021). Beyond their academic pursuits, students forged connections and collaborated across disciplinary boundaries. Study groups were formed virtually, where students from diverse majors shared strategies for coping with online coursework, managing stress, and maintaining motivation. These cross-disciplinary interactions fostered a sense of universal brotherhood and mutual support. These informal networks transcended disciplinary differences, reinforcing the idea that resilience was a collective endeavour. By pooling their knowledge, empathy, and problem-solving skills, students collectively navigated the pandemic-induced education disruptions. Their ability to draw strength from one another exemplified the power of community resilience, transcending the confines of specific fields of study.

Conclusion

This research carries substantial significance as it contributes to the existing body of literature on resilience by centring on the unique experiences of undergraduate students post-COVID-19. Understanding resilience as a multidimensional construct involving various factors such as self-awareness, relationships, problem-solving, and organisation underscores the importance of adopting a holistic approach to resilience-building interventions (Joyce et al., 2018). Resilience is indeed a broad and multidimensional concept that extends beyond individual psychological traits. While understanding resilience at a psychological level is important, it's equally essential to recognise the context in which resilience operates. Resilience is a choice, not a trait as mentioned by. Context plays a significant role in shaping resilience, as individuals navigate various socio-cultural, economic, and environmental factors that influence their ability to adapt and thrive in the face of adversity. These contextual factors can include social support networks, access to resources, cultural beliefs and practices, and systemic inequalities. Taking a holistic perspective towards resilience involves acknowledging and addressing these contextual factors, as they can profoundly impact an individual's resilience level. By understanding the complex interplay between individual characteristics and external influences, interventions, and support programs can be designed to promote resilience more comprehensively and effectively. Therefore, a nuanced understanding of resilience requires consideration of both individual psychological factors and the broader context in which resilience unfolds. This holistic perspective enables a more comprehensive approach to resilience-building that takes into account the diverse needs and challenges faced by individuals within their unique contexts.

This research was an attempt to understand how undergraduate students in Kerala have navigated the challenges brought about by the COVID-19 pandemic, emphasising their resilience. Utilising a quantitative approach and a standardised tool, the study tried to provide actionable insight for educational institutions and stakeholders, aiding in the development of strategies to support students' well-being in the evolving post-pandemic landscape. The findings are poised to shed light not only on the resilience levels of students but also to provide actionable insights for educational institutions, policymakers, and mental health professionals to craft targeted support systems. Recognising the interconnectedness of different dimensions of resilience, institutions can develop tailored support programs that address specific areas of need for students.

Implications

The resilience-building and maintenance programs can be designed for the student community and these programs can focus on enhancing self-awareness, fostering positive relationships, improving problem-solving skills, and promoting effective performance-oriented strategies. Highlighting the role of collective action and support in fostering resilience during challenging times like the COVID-19 pandemic can encourage community engagement and collaboration. Institutions can promote initiatives that encourage students to come together, support one another, and share resources to navigate shared challenges effectively. Educating students, faculty, and staff about the importance of resilience and providing resources for resilience-building can empower individuals to proactively manage challenges and setbacks. Workshops, seminars, and online resources can be developed to raise awareness about resilience and provide practical strategies for enhancing resilience in academic and personal life. Regular monitoring and evaluation of resilience-building initiatives can help institutions assess their effectiveness and make necessary adjustments. Gathering feedback from students and stakeholders can provide valuable insights into the impact of these initiatives and inform future resilience-building efforts. While reiterating, the implications of the research underscore the importance of adopting a comprehensive and proactive approach to resilience-building in educational settings, with a focus on addressing the diverse needs and challenges faced by students. By promoting resilience at individual, interpersonal, and institutional levels, educational institutions can better support students in navigating adversity and thriving in their academic and personal lives.

Limitations

The research is based on the self-reports shared by the participants and their sole perspectives have been considered without any validation. Another notable concern could be the limited sample size as the research encouraged voluntary participation. This will restrict the generalisability of the results.

Conflict of Interest

The authors declare that the research was conducted in the absence of any commercial or financial relationships that could be construed as a potential conflict of interest.

Funding

The author(s) declare that no financial support was received for the research, authorship, and/or publication of this article.

References

Ali, S., & George, A. (2021). Social inclusivity: A case study on community resilience during the Kerala flood of 2018. In *Sustainable urban architecture: Select proceedings of VALU2020* (pp. 109–131). Springer Singapore. https://doi.org/10.1007/978-981-15-9585-1_8

Ang, W. H. D., Shorey, S., Lopez, V., Chew, H. S. J., & Lau, Y. (2022). Generation Z undergraduate students' resilience during the COVID-19 pandemic: A qualitative study. *Current Psychology, 41*(11), 8132–8146. https://doi.org/10.1007/s12144-021-01830-4

Cassidy, S. (2016). The Academic Resilience Scale (ARS-30): A new multidimensional construct measure. *Frontiers in Psychology, 7*, 222168. https://doi.org/10.3389/fpsyg.2016.01787

Comin, D. A., Cruz, M., Cirera, X., Lee, K. M., & Torres, J. (2022). Technology and Resilience *(No. w29644)*. National Bureau of Economic Research. https://doi.org/10.3386/w29644

Cross, R., Dillon, K., & Greenberg, D. (2021). The secret to building resilience. *Harvard Business Review*, 1–8.

Cutter, S. L., Ash, K. D., & Emrich, C. T. (2016). Urban–rural differences in disaster resilience. *Annals of the American Association of Geographers*, *106*(6), 1236–1252. https://doi.org/10.1080/24694452.2016.1194740

Fayez, O., Ismail, H., & Aboelnagah, H. (2023). Emerging virtual communities of practice during crises: A sustainable model validating the levels of peer motivation and support. *Sustainability*, *15*(7), 5691. https://doi.org/10.3390/su15075691

Fuller-Iglesias, H., Sellars, B., & Antonucci, T. C. (2008). Resilience in old age: Social relations as a protective factor. *Research in Human Development*, *5*(3), 181–193. https://doi.org/10.1080/15427600802274043

GoK Dashboard (2022, September 09). *Official Kerala COVID-19 Statistics*. Kerala: COVID-19 Battle. https://dashboard.kerala.gov.in/covid/

Grygorenko, Z., & Naydonova, G. (2023). The concept of "resilience": history of formation and approaches to definition. *Public Administration and Law Review*, *2*, 76–88. https://doi.org/10.36690/2674-5216-2023-2-76-88

Haddadi, P., & Besharat, M. A. (2010). Resilience, vulnerability and mental health. *Procedia-Social and Behavioural Sciences*, *5*, 639–642. https://doi.org/10.1016/j.sbspro.2010.07.157

Horgan, N. (2014). *Mindfulness-Based Interventions in the Workplace. A Case Study* (Doctoral dissertation, National University of Ireland).

Joyce, S., Shand, F., Tighe, J., Laurent, S. J., Bryant, R. A., & Harvey, S. B. (2018). Road to resilience: a systematic review and meta-analysis of resilience training programmes and interventions. *British Medical Journal Open*, *8*(6), e017858. https://doi.org/10.1136/bmjopen-2017-017858

Kireeva, Z. O. (2022). Predictors of resilience and optimism in people of different ages during the SARS-COV-2 pandemic. *Scientific Bulletin of Kherson State University. Series "Psychological Sciences"*, *1*, 5–10. https://doi.org/10.32999/ksu2312-3206/2022-1-1

Linnell, M. (2014). Citizen response in crisis: Individual and collective efforts to enhance community resilience. *Human Technology*, *10*(2), 68–94. https://doi.org/10.17011/ht/urn.201411203311

Madhavan, M., Anjana, V., Mini, G.K. (2022). University students' perceptions of shifting between online and offline learning: lessons from Kerala, India. *Asian Association of Open Universities Journal*, *17*(3), 213–228. https://doi.org/10.1108/aaouj-03-2022-0031

Mashayekhi D, M. R., & Mohammadi, M. (2014). Resilience and spiritual intelligence predictors of as academic self-efficacy in urban and rural students. *Journal of School Psychology*, *3*(2), 205–225.

Morato, A. E. P., Hostalácio, S. F. S., Moura, T. P., Castro, J. P. G. B. D., Peixoto, J. M., & Moura, E. P. (2023). Resilience and spirituality of medicine students during social isolation due to the COVID-19 pandemic. *Revista Brasileira de Educação Médica*, *47*, e122.

Mowbray, D. (2008). Building resilience–an organisational cultural approach to mental health and well-being at work: a primary prevention programme. In *Employee Well-Being Support: A Workplace Resource*. West Sussex: John Wiley & Sons, 309–321. https://doi.org/10.1002/9780470773246.ch25

Mowbray, D. (2014). Strengthening personal resilience. *Management Advisory Service*, *24*, 24.

Neville, H. A., Ruedas-Gracia, N., Lee, B. A., Ogunfemi, N., Maghsoodi, A. H., Mosley, D. V., LaFromboise, T. D., & Fine, M. (2021). The public psychology for liberation training model: A call to transform the discipline. *American Psychologist*, *76*(8), 1248. https://doi.org/10.1037/amp0000887

Pattnaik, J., Nath, N., & Nath, S. (2023). Challenges to remote instruction during the pandemic: A qualitative study with primary grade teachers in India. *Early Childhood Education Journal, 51*(4), 675–684. https://doi.org/10.1007/s10643-022-01331-4

Prager, K. (2012). Collective efforts to manage cultural landscapes for resilience. In *Resilience and the Cultural Landscape. Understanding and Managing Change in Human-Shaped Environments.* Cambridge, UK: Cambridge University Press, *16*, 205–223. https://doi.org/10.1017/CBO9781139107778

Rafi, A. M., Varghese, P. R., & Kuttichira, P. (2020). The pedagogical shift during COVID-19 pandemic: Online medical education, barriers and perceptions in central Kerala. *Journal of Medical Education and Curricular Development*, *7*, 2382120520951795. https://doi.org/10.1177/2382120520951

Rahman, A. (2021). Using students' experience to derive effectiveness of COVID-19-lockdown-induced emergency online learning at undergraduate level: Evidence from Assam, India. *Higher Education for the Future*, *8*(1), 71–89. https://doi.org/10.1177/2347631120980549

Rea, L. M., & Parker, R. A. (2014). *Designing and Conducting Survey Research: A Comprehensive Guide*. John Wiley & Sons.

Roulston, A., Montgomery, L., Campbell, A., & Davidson, G. (2018). Exploring the impact of mindfulnesss on mental wellbeing, stress and resilience of undergraduate social work students. *Social Work Education*, *37*(2), 157–172. https://doi.org/10.1080/02615479.2017.1388776

Rutter, M. (2023). Resilience: Some conceptual considerations. *Social Work*, 122–127.

Salimi, N., Gere, B., Talley, W., & Irioogbe, B. (2023). College students mental health challenges: concerns and considerations in the COVID-19 pandemic. *Journal of College Student Psychotherapy*, *37*(1), 39–51. https://doi.org/10.1080/87568225.2021.1890298

Salzman, M. R. (2021). *The Falls of Rome: Crises, Resilience, and Resurgence in Late Antiquity*. Cambridge University Press.

Sojer, P., Kainbacher, S., Hüfner, K., Kemmler, G., & Deisenhammer, E. A. (2024). Trait emotional intelligence and resilience: Gender differences among university students. *Neuropsychiatrie*, *38*(1), 39–46. https://doi.org/10.1007/s40211-023-00484-x

Sun, J., & Stewart, D. (2007). Age and gender effects on resilience in children and adolescents. *International Journal of Mental Health Promotion*, *9*(4), 16–25. https://doi.org/10.1080/14623730.2007.9721845

Sundararaman, T., Muraleedharan, V. R., & Ranjan, A. (2021). Pandemic resilience and health systems preparedness: Lessons from COVID-19 for the twenty-first century. *Journal of Social and Economic Development*, *23*(Suppl 2), 290–300. https://doi.org/10.1007/s40847-020-00133-x

Svence, G., Majors, M., Majors, M., & Majors, M. (2015). Correlation of well-being with resilience and age. *Problems of Psychology in the 21st Century*, *9*(1), 45–56. https://doi.org/10.33225/ppc/15.09.45

Vinod, A., & Kini, M. K. (2022). Disaster resilience and rehabilitation in Kerala: A critical review of CARe-Kerala's housing scheme. *A System Engineering Approach to Disaster Resilience: Select Proceedings of VCDRR* 2021, 275–288. https://doi.org/10.1007/978-981-16-7397-9_20

5 Psychological After-Effects of COVID-19 among Women Survivors of Maharashtra

Pradnya Nitin Kulkarni and Vaidya Leena S. Bavadekar

Introduction

India is one of the most affected countries by the COVID-19 pandemic. During the first and second waves (from 3 January 2020 to 31 May 2021), 2,88,09,339 cases and 3,46,759 deaths were reported by the World Health Organization (2021). The highest incidence of death due to COVID-19 in India was evident in Maharashtra (Government of India, 2024), especially in the densely populated cities of Mumbai, Pune, Thane, and Nagpur. The first wave in Maharashtra extended from March 2020 to mid-February 2021, whereas the second wave was from March 2021 to May 2021. The Pune district was worst affected during both waves, with 10,17,154 cases and 12,507 fatalities (1.23 per cent) (Shil et al., 2022).

Pandemic and Psychological Distress

During the first and second waves, the novel nature of the virus, fear of getting an infection, and circumstances such as lockdown, quarantine, hospitalisation, changing symptoms, inadequate treatments, etc., posed significant psychological distress in Indian society (Chamaa et al., 2021; Joshi, 2021; Sharma et al., 2022). It was reported that being diagnosed positive on the COVID-19 test was a significant trauma (Zheng et al., 2021). Along with the illness-related fear, being quarantined for a minimum of 2 weeks, either at home or at quarantine centres was a very unusual psychosocial stressor (Brooks et al., 2020) that constrained the most needed social and family support at that time. During the initial phases of the pandemic, stigma against infected individuals added to the trauma of COVID-19 (Bhatnagar et al., 2021; Singh & Subedi, 2020; Galicia, 2021). One of the significant effects of the COVID-19 period was job loss and financial crunches (Nag, 2020). Socio-economic factors were essential contributors to the perceived stress of COVID-19. Literature shows that anxiety symptoms were associated with socio-economic class, and the most affected group was that of homemakers (Rai et al., 2021; Das, 2020).

The cumulative effect of pandemic-related stressors is evident in the mental health of the patients. Mental health comorbidities such as anxiety, depression, acute stress reactions, and post-traumatic stress were commonly reported among

DOI: 10.4324/9781003517313-6

COVID-19 patients (Dar et al., 2021). Various studies also indicate that the mental health impact of COVID-19 infection was long-lasting and sustained even after the recovery of the physical symptoms. Commonly observed symptoms among survivors were anxiety, depression, sleeplessness, and post-traumatic stress disorder (PTSD) (Wu et al., 2020; Mei, 2021; Mazza et al., 2022).

The COVID-19 pandemic is considered a traumatic event due to the widespread feelings of despondency, uncertainty, and anxiety it has caused at both individual and community levels. These feelings are driven by fears of contracting a highly infectious and potentially life-threatening disease. So, individuals who have contracted the virus or lost a close relative unexpectedly to the illness may perceive the experience as traumatic. Research shows that globally, the presence of PTSD symptoms is evident among certain groups during the COVID-19 era (Sun et al.,2020; Wu et al., 2020; Mei, 2021; Mazza et al., 2022) and COVID-19 survivors are the most vulnerable group to develop mental health problems like PTSD (Dar et al., 2021).

Women and Pandemic Distress

Gender is an essential social determinant of health and mental health (Connor et al., 2020). Literature shows that women were at higher risk for mental health issues such as anxiety (Farhane-Medina, 2022), depression (WHO, 2023), and PTSD (Gradus, 2017) than men. Literature also shows the aggravated psychological impact of the pandemic on females (Gopal et al., 2020). The stressors like the increased traditional expectations of caregiving, low family support, domestic violence, and fear of infection to self and family members increased mental health vulnerability among Indian women during the pandemic (Joshi, 2021; Huq, 2021). Literature reported that female patients infected with COVID-19 had experienced more significant distress than males (Dar, 2021; Wu et al., 2020; Connor et al., 2020). Studies among women survivors showed that women experienced higher mood symptoms and impaired quality of life (Lindahl et al., 2022) and also higher post-traumatic stress symptoms (Wu et al., 2022) than males. Longitudinal research with this respect reported psychological after-effects such as pathological fatigue and depression among COVID-19 survivors 6 months and 12 months after the recovery. Still, interestingly, declining depression was evident for females, and a reverse trend was apparent for males (Mazza et al., 2022). Thus, gender differences were noticeable in distress coping, which is well supported by the literature (Helgeson, 2011). According to Matud (2004), women exhibited higher somatic symptoms and psychological distress. They were higher on emotions-focused and avoidant coping styles and lower on rational and detachment styles. Concerning COVID-19 stressors, gender differences are also evident in risk perception and coping mechanisms (Rana et al., 2021).

Considering the high vulnerability of women to mental health problems, it is essential to study the long-term mental health effects of COVID-19 among women. There are very few studies in the Indian setup that explore the psychological after-effects of COVID-19 among female survivors. Also, it is essential to understand these psychological after-effects in the light of social and demographic contributors, which is scantly represented in the Indian literature. Thus, the current study explores psychological after-effects and their socio-demographic contributors. As the urban setup of Pune was highly affected during the pandemic, research focused on women in the urban area of Pune.

Purpose of the Study

The study tries to explore the psychological after-effects of COVID-19 among Maharashtra's women survivors. It also intends to determine the role of socio-demographic factors in the psychological after-effects.

Method

Research Design

The study adopted a cross-cultural survey research design.

Sample

It was a purposive sample of 304 women aged 18–65 (mean 44) from Pune, Maharashtra, India. The study included patients infected during the first and second waves from March 2020 to March 2021. Figure 5.1 shows the frequency distribution across socio-demographic variables. It shows that most women, nearly 60%,

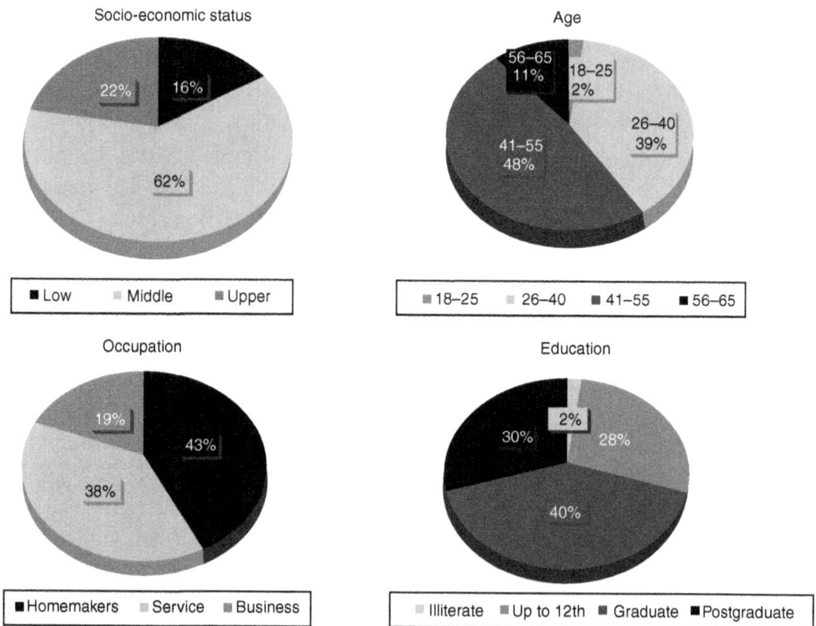

Figure 5.1 Frequency distribution across socio-demographic variables.

were from the middle and upper–middle-class. Lower and upper-class representation is comparatively low, 18% and 22%, respectively. Age-wise frequency distribution shows a higher representation of middle-aged women between 41 and 55. The frequency of working women is slightly higher (57%) than that of homemakers (43%). And, the majority of the women (70%) were graduates and above.

Inclusion Criteria

1 One month to 12 months after detecting the significant symptoms of COVID-19.
2 Patients who were recovered from COVID-19.
3 Patients who were discharged from hospital and quarantine centres.

Exclusion Criteria

1 Active symptomatic women patients.
2 Confirmation of a positive COVID-19 report within less than 1 month.

Procedure

To collect the data at the outset the patients' contact numbers were obtained from the selected hospitals and quarantine centres. As the data collection happened during the lockdown phase, it was collected telephonically by trained female surveyors in April 2021. The informed consent was obtained from each participant and they were briefed about the objective of the research. Confidentiality was assured, and the right to quit the research process was informed. The general information questionnaire and traumatic stress disorder checklist for DSM 5 were administered verbally, and the surveyors noted participants' responses. The participants' identifying information was removed from the data files to preserve confidentiality.

Measures

The following tools were used.

General Information Questionnaire (GIQ): The GIQ includes socio-demographics and details related to the duration of COVID-19 infection, symptoms and reactions of family members, support by family members, etc. It included two open-ended questions:

1 How was your mental status reacting to COVID-19 infection?
2 How did you cope with this life event?

Traumatic Stress Disorder Checklist for DSM 5 (PCL-5) (National Centre for PTSD, 2016): This measures current distress levels and trauma symptoms. This tool is open source with good psychometric properties: internal consistency ($\alpha = 0.94$), test–retest reliability ($r = 0.82$), and convergent ($rs = 0.74$–0.85) and discriminant validity ($rs = 0.31$–0.60) (Blevins et al., 2015). The PCL-5 is a 5-point rating scale with 21 items, scored from 0 to 4; a score of 2 and above for each item was considered significant for clinical inquiry. It measures intrusion symptoms, avoidance, negative changes in feelings and mood, arousal, and reactivity. According to PCL-5, the critical value of 31 and above is interpreted as clinically significant to consider PTSD diagnosis (National Center for PTSD, 2016). The tool was translated into the Marathi language. Three experts rated the PCL items for translation accuracy on a 5-point scale. Items with a mean score of 4 and above were retained, and a few items with a mean score below 4 were modified according to the expert's suggestions.

Data Analysis

The questionnaire's quantitative data and PCL-5 were analysed using SPSS version 22. Frequencies, descriptive statistics, chi-square, and Spearman rank correlation were calculated.

Results

Descriptive Statistics of PCL

Figure 5.2 indicates distribution of PCL scores across sample which is positively skewed. Table 5.1 shows the descriptive statistics of scores of total PCL and its four subdomains: total avoidance, negative feelings and mood, total arousal, and adaptability. The data indicate low mean and median values for Total PCL and all domains.

The data in Table 5.2 show that the majority of the participants (57.4%) reported milder psychological distress. A clinically significant level of distress is observed in 1.9% of the participants.

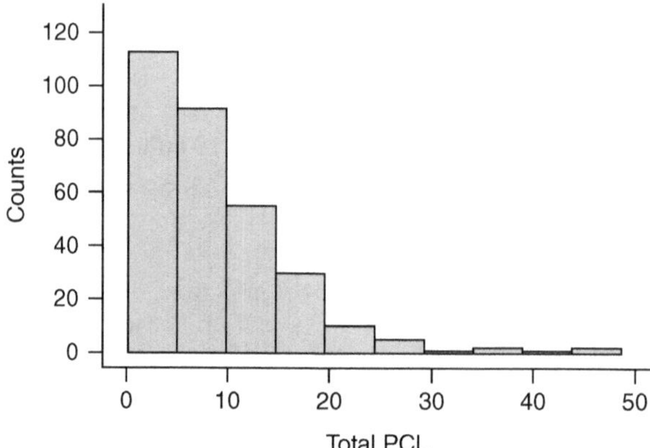

Figure 5.2 Distribution of PCL scores of COVID-19 women survivors.

Table 5.1 Descriptive statistics of PCL ($N = 304$)

	Total intrusion	*Total avoidance*	*Total negative feelings and mood*	*Total arousal and reactivity*	*Total PCL*
Mean	2.08	1.92	1.67	3.51	9.19
Median	1.00	1.50	1.00	3.00	8.00
Std. Deviation	2.53	1.85	2.62	2.89	7.82

Table 5.2 Level of psychological distress across the sample ($N = 304$)

Particular	*Score range*	*Sample*
No distress	0	8.3%
Mild level distress	01–10	57.4%
Moderate level distress	11–20	27.2%
Moderately high-level distress	21–30	5.2%
Clinically significant distress (PTSD)	31 and above	1.9%
Total		100%

Item-wise analysis in Table 5.3 shows that the most frequently observed stress symptoms were 'being super alert about COVID-19' (mean = 2.06; SD = 1.59) and 'avoiding external reminders of COVID-19 illness' (mean = 1.38; SD = 1.49).

Psychological After-Effects Across Socio-Demographic Variables

The psychological after-effects were analysed across socio-demographic variables, such as socio-economic status (assessed based on annual family income) and occupation, education, age, and circumstantial factors such as isolation arrangements, recovery duration, etc. Since the PCL score distribution does not conform to the assumptions of normality, the non-parametric Kruskal–Wallis test was used for analysis.

Psychological After-Effects Across Socio-Economic Status

Table 5.4 shows that the H value is significant only for 'intrusion symptoms'; Chi-Square value x^2 (df = 2, $N = 304$) = 6.14, $p < 0.05$ indicates that 'intrusion symptoms' differ across socio-economic classes. However, there is no significant difference in total PCL and other subdomains across socio-economic statuses.

Table 5.5 shows that the lower class most frequently displays 'intrusion symptoms', followed by the middle and upper classes.

Table 5.3 Descriptive statistics of PCL item-wise ($N = 304$)

Item No.	*PCL items*	*Mean*	*SD*
1	Repeated, disturbing, unwanted memories of COVID-19	0.86	1.083
2	Repeated disturbing dreams about COVID-19	0.13	0.427
3	The feeling of repetitive occurrence of COVID-19	0.33	0.71
4	Upset with reminders of COVID-19 incidence	0.5	0.84
5	Physical reactions like palpitations or sweating with reminders of COVID-19	0.26	0.62
6	Avoiding thinking/memories of COVID-19	0.56	0.881
7	Avoiding external reminders of COVID-19	1.38	1.496
8	Trouble in remembering COVID-19 illness-related things	0.16	0.509
9	Negative feelings about self or situation	0.34	0.732
10	Blaming others and self for the situation	0.17	0.502
11	Strong negative feelings (fear, horror, anger)	0.32	0.75
12	Loss of interest in previously liked activities	0.21	0.663
13	Feeling distant or cut-off from others	0.28	0.716
14	Trouble in experiencing positive emotions	0.22	0.698
15	Irritable behaviour, angry outburst	0.42	0.784
16	Making harm to self or others	0.08	0.403
17	Super alert about COVID-19	2.06	1.59
18	Feeling jumpy, startled	0.2	0.545
19	Difficulty in concentrating	0.34	0.766
20	Difficulty in sleeping	0.43	0.931
21	Effect on daily routine	0.94	1.187

Table 5.4 PCL domain and subdomain differences across socio-economic status (df = 2)

	Total intrusion	*Total avoidance*	*Total negative feeling mood*	*Total arousal and reactivity*	*Total PCL*
H value	5.77	2.33	0.034	5.16	3.79
Chi-square	6.136	2.447	0.394	5.261	3.801
Asymptotic significance	0.047	0.294	0.821	0.072	0.149

Note: Kruskal–Wallis test.

Table 5.5 Mean ranks of intrusion symptoms across SES groups

Economic status		*N*	*Mean rank*
Total intrusion	Low	49	184.12
	Middle	187	151.92
	Upper	68	148.83
	Total	304	

Table 5.6 PCL domain and subdomain differences across occupations (df = 2)

	Total intrusion	*Total avoidance*	*Total negative feeling/mood*	*Total arousal and reactivity*	*Total PCL*
H value	6.67	1.44	1.77	8.42	7.60
Chi-square	7.093	1.514	2.035	8.590	7.632
Asymptotic significance	0.029	0.469	0.361	0.014	0.022

Note: Kruskal–Wallis test.

Table 5.7 Mean ranks of significant symptom domains across occupation

Occupation	*N*	*Mean ranks*		
		Intrusion	*Arousal and reactivity*	*Total PCL*
Home makers	130	169.73	170.48	170.35
Service	116	152.61	153.92	152.92
Business	58	134.31	129.94	132.25

Psychological After-Effects Across Occupation

Table 5.6 shows that the *H* value is significant for 'intrusion symptoms', 'arousal', and 'reactivity symptoms', and total PCL score. Chi-square value indicates that intrusion symptoms x^2 (df = 2, N = 304) = 7.09, $p < 0.05$; arousal and reactivity symptoms x^2 (df = 2, N = 304) = 8.6, $p < 0.05$) and total PCL scores x^2 (df = 2, N = 304) = 7.63, $p < 0.05$ differ across occupation. Whereas avoidance symptoms and negative mood symptoms do not differ across occupations.

Table 5.7 shows that homemakers most frequently experienced 'distress symptoms', 'specifically intrusion', 'arousal', and 'reactivity symptoms'. It is followed by women engaged in service and business showing the least-frequent symptoms respective to subdomains and total stress symptoms. No significant differences in distress symptoms were found across women's education and age groups.

Psychological After-Effects Across Isolation Arrangements

Women survivors underwent three types of isolation arrangements: home quarantine, quarantine centres, and hospitals. Table 5.8 shows PCL score differences across these three groups.

Table 5.8 shows that the *H* value is significant only for intrusion symptoms; Chi-square value x^2 (df = 2, N = 304) = 12.66, $p < 0.05$ indicates that intrusion symptoms differ across isolation arrangements. Whereas total PCL, avoidance symptoms, negative mood, arousal, and reactivity, these distress symptoms do not differ across isolation arrangements.

Table 5.8 PCL domain and subdomain differences across isolation arrangements (df = 2)

	Total intrusion	*Total avoidance*	*Total negative feelings & mood*	*Total arousal and reactivity*	*Total PCL*
H value	11.91	.10	1.5	0.38	1.86
Chi-square	12.66	.107	1.717	0.392	1.87
Asymptotic significance	0.002	0.948	0.424	0.822	0.39

Note: Kruskal–Wallis test.

Table 5.9 Mean ranks of significant symptom domains across isolation arrangement

		n	*Mean rank*
Total intrusion	Home	174	141.05
	Quarantine centre	48	179.31
	Hospital	82	174.91
	Total	304	

Table 5.9 shows that the women isolated in quarantine centres had the highest PCL scores, followed by hospital-admitted women. Whereas home quarantine women experienced the most minor distress, as indicated by their PCL scores. Women isolated in quarantine centres were high on the following symptoms; 'Unwanted upsetting memories', 'reliving trauma', 'avoiding trauma-related thoughts' and 'feelings', and 'avoiding reminders of the trauma'.

Correlation Between Distress Symptoms and Duration of Recovery

Spearman rank difference correlation was calculated between 'distress symptoms' and 'duration of recovery'. There is a significant positive but low correlation between the duration of total symptom recovery of COVID-19 and total PCL ($\rho = 0.221$; $p < 0.01$), intrusion symptoms ($\rho = 0.142$; $p < 0.05$), avoidance symptoms ($\rho = 0.171$; $p < 0.01$), negative mood ($\rho = 0.219$; $p < 0.01$), and arousal and reactivity ($\rho = 0.166$; $p < 0.01$).

Discussion

In India, the limited medical infrastructure and the large population made dealing with COVID-19 not only a medical emergency but also a very stressful and traumatic experience. Literature showed that the pandemic effects were predominantly high for women (Gopal et al., 2020). Higher distress was reported by female patients suffering from COVID-19 symptoms than males (Dar, 2021; Wu et al., 2020; Connor et al., 2020). In general, the literature indicated that in response to stressful situations, women were prone to mental health disturbances (Matud, 2004) like anxiety (Farhane-Medina, 2022), depression (WHO, 2023), and PTSD (Chandana et al., 2023; Gradus, 2017). Consistent with the literature, even Indian studies showed a high incidence of PTSD among COVID-19 patients (Dar et al., 2021). In this context, the current study explored the long-term effect of COVID-19 infection on women survivors. Also, the study examined the underlying socio-demographic variables that contributed to the distress symptoms and its recovery.

The meta-analytic studies among COVID-19 survivors representing 13 nations from Europe, the USA, the Middle East, and Asia Pacific countries showed the prevalence of PTSD to be 16% (95% confidence interval: 9%–23%) (Nagarajan et al., 2022). A study conducted in North India on patients during hospitalisation also suggests a 25.21% prevalence of PTSD among COVID survivors using PCL-5 (Dar et al., 2021). However, using the same scale and cut-off scores for women samples, the current study suggested that 1.9% of women developed clinically significant symptoms of PTSD as measured after 1–12 months. Though not clinically significant, most women reported mild distress, and approximately one-third showed moderate to moderately severe distress. The global as well as Indian epidemiology estimates about PTSD in the general population showed a high prevalence among women (Chandana et al., 2023; Gradus, 2017). However, compared to the global prevalence of PTSD, prevalence in India is significantly low (0.2%) (Chandna et al., 2023). The current findings align with this study, indicating a low rate of PTSD among women survivors despite reports of mild to moderate subclinical distress due to COVID-19 illness. Studies have explained the phenomenon of low prevalence of PTSD among Indian women to socio-cultural factors (Chandna et al., 2023). Traditionally, Indian society is collectivistic, valuing cohesiveness, interdependence, and support among family, friends, and society (Verma, 2020; Kordyban et al., 2016). Traditional collectivist cultural values and other resilience-promoting cultural health factors like family and social support were noted to promote resilience and reduce the risk for PTSD (Oakley et al., 2021). During the COVID-19 pandemic, socio-cultural factors served as protection for mental health (Mahamid & Bdier, 2021; Das, 2020; Jia et al., 2021; Li et al., 2021) even played an important role in post-traumatic growth (Joy et al., 2023). In the current study, 96% of women reported acceptance and support from family members and different types of support from society, which might have helped women. During the telephonic interview, women reported that venting distress to friends, family members, and relatives reduced the traumatic effect of COVID-19.

Among COVID-19 survivors, the fear of recurrence of COVID-19 was commonly evident (Dar et al., 2021). The current study also reported the 'super alertness about illness', which might be associated with fear of the recurrence of COVID-19. Another symptom of avoiding external reminders of COVID-19 illnesses was the most commonly reported reaction. Media played an important role in aggravating the anxiety related to COVID-19 (Bendau et al., 2021; Liu & Liu, 2020). During the interview, women reported that they had stopped watching COVID-19-related news. Thus, avoidance worked as a helpful coping strategy for distress management.

The available research also highlights the impact of socio-demographic variables across the distress symptoms (Rai et al., 2021; Das, 2020). Socio-economic factors are the major determinants concerning resources available for COVID-19 challenges. Loss of jobs and financial crunches were among the major effects of the COVID-19 period (Nag, 2020). In the current study, the effect of low socio-economic resources on the aggravation of psychological distress was evident

Similarly, homemakers seemed to be at higher risk of psychological distress as compared to working women. For working women, better availability of resources, engagement in activities, and higher social networks seemed to minimise the effect of trauma.

One of the stressful factors for COVID-19 survivors was quarantine arrangements. The negative psychological impact of quarantine during the morbidity phase, as well as its long-term psychological effects, were reported in the literature (Brooks et al., 2020). A study in the Indian setup showed that 71% of the discharged COVID-19 patients reported quarantine-related stigma (Bhatnagar, 2021). In India, quarantine centres were launched during the first and second waves to prevent disease transmission. Patients found positive on the COVID-19 test sought admission to the quarantine centres. It seemed that the experience of these quarantine centres added to the trauma. Comparatively, home quarantine women felt safe and were less traumatised.

The study also showed that psychological distress was associated with the duration of illness symptoms. Thus, the prolonged and chronic nature of illness is directly associated with psychological distress. Longitudinal studies showed a declining trend of PTSD symptoms along duration after the stressful life event (Mazza et al., 2022); however, the cross-sectional differences related to distress across 3-, 6-, 9-, and 12-month periods were not evident in the current study.

Thus, the study highlighted that socio-demographic factors contributed significantly to the trauma symptoms of the women survivors. Women from lower socio-economic classes, homemakers, and those who were admitted to quarantine centres found this post-traumatic recovery hard. Family support and social support seemed to have worked as protective factors against COVID-19 distress among women survivors.

Conclusion

This study attempted to explore the psychological after-effects among women with COVID-19 survivors in India. It attempted to investigate the role of socio-demographic variables in the aggravation of these effects. Findings showed mild to moderate subclinical distress is evident among COVID-19 women survivors, but the clinical prevalence of PTSD in the current sample is comparatively lower than reported in other studies. Among socio-demographic variables, women from lower socio-economic class women, homemakers, and those who were isolated in quarantine centres showed higher distress symptoms even after the recovery from COVID-19. Family and social support were reported to be protective factors against the trauma stress of COVID-19 infection.

Implication

This study confirms the prolonged presence of comorbid mental health issues that persist with health conditions like COVID-19. There is a need to recognise these comorbid mental health conditions by health workers and family members and extend help to manage them. Also, during follow-up check-ups along with health parameters, the importance of assessing mental health parameters is implicated in this study. The study showed that though mild to moderate subclinical distress is evident among COVID-19 women survivors, the clinical prevalence of PTSD in the current sample is comparatively lower than reported in the literature. One of the reasons could be family and social resources, which could have buffered trauma distress. This implies that strengthening personal and social resources is essential to endure illness stressors. Building psychosocial resources for women is most important for those who are at risk; that is, those from lower socio-economic classes, homemakers who have a comorbidity of mental illness, and those previously traumatised. Healthcare systems need to address these issues while treating health conditions. Special efforts to reduce stigma by social and health agencies are required not only for COVID-19 but also for related health and mental health conditions. Thus, research implies the need for attention to psychological after-effects and their management for women patients by healthcare facilities and society.

Acknowledgements

This paper is a part of the survey by Sharada Shakti; Maharashtra unit of Shakti—A National movement for women. We acknowledge the support of Dr Sangeeta Kale, President, Sharada Shakti, and Mrs Manisha Kulkarni, Secretary, Sharada Shakti, for conducting this survey. We also acknowledge the team leaders Dr Apoorva Sangoram, Dr Maithili Nesargi-Naik, Dr Ankita Badgujar, Dr Aishwarya Ranade, Mrs Mrudula Arjunwadkar under whose guidance a team of 35 surveyors collected data. We also acknowledge the contribution of Dr Pramod Dhumal, Mrs Simantini, Vaze, Dr Indira Ujagare, Dr Manasi Deshpande, Aruna Joshu, Mrudul Shigurkar, Dr Priyamvada Herlekar, Dr Rajashree Kashalkar, Dr Manisha Khaladkar, Dr Himani Godbole, Sneha Joshi. We also acknowledge Priti Bhat and her team provided support for statistical analysis.

Funding

NGO Sharada Shakti, Maharashtra unit of Shakti—A National movement for women funded the project.

Conflict of Interest

The authors declare that they have no conflicts of interest.

Data Availability

The data supporting this study's findings are available on request from the corresponding author. The data are not publicly available because it contains information that could compromise the privacy of research participants.

References

Ahmed, H., Patel, K., Greenwood, D. C., Halpin, S., Lewthwaite, P., Salawu, A., ... & Sivan, M. (2020). Long-term clinical outcomes in survivors of severe acute respiratory syndrome (SARS) and Middle East respiratory syndrome coronavirus (MERS) outbreaks after hospitalisation or ICU admission: A systematic review and meta-analysis. *Journal of Rehabilitation Medicine*, *52*(5), 1–11.

American Psychiatric Association. (2022). Posttraumatic stress disorder. In *Diagnostic and statistical manual of mental disorders* (5th ed., Text rev.).

Bendau, A., Petzold, M. B., Pyrkosch, L., Mascarell Maricic, L., Betzler, F., Rogoll, J., Grobe, J., Strohle, A., & Plag, J. (2021). Associations between COVID-19 related media consumption and symptoms of anxiety, depression and COVID-19 related fear in the general population in Germany. *European Archives of Psychiatry and Clinical Neuroscience*, *271*, 283–291. https://doi.org/10.1007/s00406-021-01290-8

Bhatnagar, S., Kumar, S., Rathore, P., Sarma, R., Malhotra, R. K., Choudhary, N., Thankachan, A., Haokip, N., Singh, S., Pandit, V.S., Ratre, B., Mohan, A., Lorenz, K., & Guleria, R. (2021). Surviving COVID-19 is half the battle; living life with perceived stigma is other half: a cross-sectional study. *Indian Journal of Psychological Medicine*, *43*(5), 428–435. https://doi.org/10.1177/02537176211029331

Blevins, C. A., Weathers, F. W., Davis, M. T., Witte, T. K., & Domino, J. L. (2015). The posttraumatic stress disorder checklist for DSM-5 (PCL-5): Development and initial psychometric evaluation. *Journal of Traumatic Stress*, *28*(6), 489–498. https://doi.org/10.1002/jts.22059

Brooks, S. K., Webster, R. K., Smith, L. E., Woodland, L., Wessely, S., Greenberg, N., & Rubin, G. J. (2020). The psychological impact of quarantine and how to reduce it: A rapid review of the evidence. *The Lancet*, *395*(10227), 912–920. https://doi.org/10.1016/S0140-6736(20)30460-8

Chamaa, F., Bahmad, H. F., Darwish, B., Kobeissi, J. M., Hoballah, M., Nassif, S. B., Ghandour, Y., Saliba, J.P., Lawand, N., & Abou-Kheir, W. (2021). PTSD in the COVID-19 era. *Current Neuropharmacology*, *19*(12), 2164. https://doi.org/10.2174%2F1570159X19666210113152954

Chandna, A. S., Suhas, S., Patley, R., Dinakaran, D., Manjunatha, N., Rao, G. N., Gururaj, G., Varghese, M., & Benegal, V. (2023). Exploring the enigma of low prevalence of posttraumatic stress disorder in India. *Indian Journal of Psychiatry*, *65*(12), 1254–1260. https://doi.org10.4103/indianjpsychiatry.indianjpsychiatry_830_23

Connor, J., Madhavan, S., Mokashi, M., Amanuel, H., Johnson, N. R., Pace, L. E., & Bartz, D. (2020). Health risks and outcomes that disproportionately affect women during the Covid-19 pandemic: A review. *Social Science & Medicine*, *266*, 113364. https://doi.org/10.1016/j.socscimed.2020.113364

Dar, S. A., Dar, M. M., Sheikh, S., Haq, I., Azad, A. M. U. D., Mushtaq, M., Shah, N., & Wani, Z. A. (2021). Psychiatric comorbidities among COVID-19 survivors in North

India: A cross-sectional study. *Journal of Education and Health Promotion, 10*, 1–9. https://doi.org/10.4103%2Fjehp.jehp_119_21

Das, S. (2020). Mental health and psychosocial aspects of COVID-19 in India: The challenges and responses. *Journal of Health Management, 22*(2), 197–205. https://doi.org/10.1177/0972063420935544

Farhane-Medina, N. Z., Luque, B., Tabernero, C., & Castillo-Mayén, R. (2022). Factors associated with gender and sex differences in anxiety prevalence and comorbidity: A systematic review. *Science Progress, 105*(4), 1–30. https://doi.org/10.1177/00368504221135469

Galica, J., Liu, Z., Kain, D., Merchant, S., Booth, C., Koven, R., Brundage, M., & Haase, K. R. (2021). Coping during COVID-19: A mixed methods study of older cancer survivors. *Supportive Care in Cancer, 29*, 3389–3398. https://doi.org/10.1007/s00520-021-05992-6

Gopal, A., Sharma, A. J., & Subramanyam, M. A. (2020). Dynamics of psychological responses to COVID-19 in India: A longitudinal study. *PLOS One, 15*(10), e0240650. https://doi.org/10.1371/journal.pone.0240650

Government of India. (2024). *COVID-19 State-Wise Status* Retrieved on 3rd April 2024, from www.mygov.in/corona-data/covid19-statewise-status/

Gradus, J. L. (2017). Prevalence and prognosis of stress disorders: A review of the epidemiologic literature. *Clinical Epidemiology*, 251–260.

Helgeson, V. S. (2011). Gender, stress, and coping. In Folkman, S. (Ed.), *The Oxford Handbook of Stress, Health, and Coping* (pp. 63–85). Oxford University Press.

Huq, M., Das, T., Devakumar, D., Daruwalla, N., & Osrin, D. (2021). Intersectional tension: A qualitative study of the effects of the COVID-19 response on Survivors of violence against women in urban India. *BMJ Open, 11*(9), e050381. https://doi.org/10.1136/bmjopen-2021-050381

Jia, Z., Xu, S., Zhang, Z., Cheng, Z., Han, H., Xu, H., Wang, M., Zhang, H., Zhou, Y., & Zhou, Z. (2021). Association between mental health and community support in lockdown communities during the COVID-19 pandemic: Evidence from rural China. *Journal of Rural Studies, 82*, 87–97. https://doi.org/10.1016/j.jrurstud.2021.01.015

Joshi, A. (2021). COVID-19 pandemic in India: Through psycho-social lens. *Journal of Social and Economic Development, 23*(Suppl 2), 414–437. https://doi.org/10.1007/s40847-020-00136-8

Joy, L. K., Kunjumon, L. E., Anil, A., Jaisankar, M., Fariha, A., Naufal, N. Z., Santosh, S.P., Kallazgi, A., & Tan, C. S. (2023). The roles of social support, family support, coping strategies, and financial safety in posttraumatic growth among COVID-19 survivors in Kerala. *Current Psychology*, 1–5. https://doi.org/10.1007/s12144-023-05175-y

Kordyban, T., Hicks, R., & Bahr, M. (2016). Understanding post-colonial India's culture. *Indian Culture and Work Organisations in Transition*, 76.

Li, F., Luo, S., Mu, W., Li, Y., Ye, L., Zheng, X., Xu., B., Ding, Y., Ling, P., Zhou, M., & Chen, X. (2021). Effects of sources of social support and resilience on the mental health of different age groups during the COVID-19 pandemic. *BMC Psychiatry, 21*, 1–14. https://doi.org/10.1186/s12888-020-03012-1

Lindahl, A., Aro, M., Reijula, J., Mäkelä, M. J., Ollgren, J., Puolanne, M., ... & Vasankari, T. (2022). Women report more symptoms and impaired quality of life: a survey of Finnish COVID-19 survivors. *Infectious Diseases, 54*(1), 53–62.

Liu, C., & Liu, Y. (2020). Media exposure and anxiety during COVID-19: The mediation effect of media vicarious traumatization. *International Journal of Environmental Research and Public Health, 17*(13), 4720. https://doi.org/10.3390/ijerph17134720

Mahamid, F. A., & Bdier, D. The association between positive religious coping, perceived stress, and depressive symptoms during the spread of coronavirus (COVID-19) among a sample of adults in Palestine: A cross-sectional study. *Journal of Religion and Health 60*, 34–49 (2021). https://doi.org/10.1007/s10943-020-01121-5

Matud, M. P. (2004). Gender differences in stress and coping styles. *Personality and Individual Differences*, *37*(7), 1401–1415.

Mazza, M. G., Palladini, M., De Lorenzo, R., Bravi, B., Poletti, S., Furlan, R., & Benedetti, F. (2022). One-year mental health outcomes in a cohort of COVID-19 survivors. *Journal of Psychiatric Research*, *145*, 118–124. https://doi.org/10.1016/j.jpsychires.2021.11.031

Mei, Q., Wang, F., Bryant, A., Wei, L., Yuan, X., & Li, J. (2021). Mental health problems among COVID-19 survivors in Wuhan, China. *World Psychiatry*, *20*(1), 139. https://doi.org/10.1002%2Fwps.20829

Nag, A. (2020). India jobless rate swells above 23% amid coronavirus lockdown, survey shows. *The Economic Times*, 7 April 2020. https://economictimes.indiatimes.com/jobs/india-jobless-rate-swells-above-23-amid-coronavirus-lockdown-survey-shows/articleshow/75023958.cms?utm_source=contentofinterest&utm_medium=text&utm_campaign=cppst

Nagarajan, R., Krishnamoorthy, Y., Basavarachar, V., & Dakshinamoorthy, R. (2022). Prevalence of post-traumatic stress disorder among survivors of severe COVID-19 infections: A systematic review and meta-analysis. *Journal of Affective Disorders*, *299*, 52–59. https://doi.org/10.1016/j.jad.2021.11.040

National Centre for PTSD. (2016). PTSD Checklist for DSM-5 (PCL-5). Retrieved from www.ptsd.va.gov/professional/ assessment/adult-sr/ptsd-checklist.asp

Oakley, L. D., Kuo, W. C., Kowalkowski, J. A., & Park, W. (2021). Meta-analysis of cultural influences in trauma exposure and PTSD prevalence rates. *Journal of Transcultural Nursing*, *32*(4), 412–424. https://doi.org/10.1177/1043659621993909

Rai, S. R., Sugreev, D. A., Pradhyuman, T., Mandal, S. D., & Chakraborthy, G. S. (2021). A cross-sectional observational study on impact of COVID-19 pandemic on mental health and quality of life in different socioeconomic groups in India. *International Journal of Pharmaceutical Sciences Review and Research*, *68*(2), 120–123. http://dx.doi.org/10.47583/ijpsrr.2021.v68i02.018

Rana, I. A., Bhatti, S. S., Aslam, A. B., Jamshed, A., Ahmad, J., & Shah, A. A. (2021). COVID-19 risk perception and coping mechanisms: Does gender make a difference? *International Journal of Disaster Risk Reduction*, *55*, 102096.

Sharma, S., Joseph, J., Dhandapani, M., Varghese, A., Radha, K., Mathews, E., & Varkey, B. P. (2022). COVID-19 and psychological distress among the general population of India: Meta-analysis of observational studies. *Indian Journal of Community Medicine*, *47*(2), 160–165. http://dx.doi.org/10.4103/ijcm.ijcm_1365_21

Shil, P., Atre, N. M., & Tandale, B. V. (2022). Epidemiological findings for the first and second waves of COVID-19 pandemic in Maharashtra, India. *Spatial and Spatio-Temporal Epidemiology*, *41*, 100507. https://doi.org/10.1016/j.sste.2022.100507

Singh, R., & Subedi, M. (2020). COVID-19 and stigma: Social discrimination towards frontline healthcare providers and COVID-19 recovered patients in Nepal. *Asian Journal of Psychiatry*, *53*, 102222. https://doi.org/10.1016%2Fj.ajp.2020.102222

Sun, L., Sun, Z., Wu, L., Zhu, Z., Zhang, F., Shang, Z., ... & Liu, W. (2020). Prevalence and risk factors of acute posttraumatic stress symptoms during the COVID-19 outbreak in Wuhan, China. *MedRxiv*, *10*(2020.03), 06–20032425.

Verma, J. (2020). Collectivism in the cultural perspective: The Indian scene. *Latest Contributions to Cross-Cultural Psychology,* 228–241, Routledge.

World Health Organization. (2021, May 31). WHO COVID-19 Dashboard https://covid19.who.int/region/searo/country/in

World Health Organization. (2023, June 15). Factsheet-Depressive disorders www.who.int/news-room/fact-sheets/detail/depression

Wu, C., Hu, X., Song, J., Yang, D., Xu, J., Cheng, ... & Du, C. (2020). Mental health status and related influencing factors of COVID-19 survivors in Wuhan, China. *Clinical and Translational Medicine*, *10*(2), e52. https://doi.org/10.1002/ctm2.52.

Wu, K. K., Lee, D., Sze, A. M., Ng, V. N., Cho, V. W., Cheng, J. P., ... & Tsang, O. T. (2022). Posttraumatic stress, anxiety, and depression in COVID-19 survivors. *East Asian Archives of Psychiatry*, *32*(1), 5–10.

Zheng, J., Morstead, T., Sin, N., Klaiber, P., Umberson, D., Kamble, S., & DeLongis, A. (2021). Psychological distress in North America during COVID-19: The role of pandemic-related stressors. *Social Science & Medicine*, *270*, 113687. https://doi.org/10.1016/j.socscimed.2021.113687

6 Browsing to Worrying in Post-COVID-19 Era

Quantifying the Links between Internet Addiction, Cyberchondria, and Health Anxiety in Emerging Adults of North-East India

Banani Basistha and Kangkan Bhuyan

Introduction

The internet has become a necessity in daily life, acting as the primary source of information, communication, and maintaining relationships with others. This dependence is further fuelled by the constant connectivity offered by modern technology, making the internet an indispensable tool in today's fast-paced world. There is growing concern about the rise in internet addiction (IA), cyberchondria, and health worries, particularly in emerging adults. According to Jeffrey Arnett, emerging adults are those who are in their late teens and lead to adulthood, comprising 18–29 years (Arnett, 2000; Arnett et al., 2014). Emerging adulthood is a period which can be considered the age of possibilities, instability, identity exploration, self-focus, and a sense of being in between adolescence and adulthood (Arnett, 2000; Arnett et al., 2014). Increasing internet dependency among emerging adults can aggravate cyberchondria in which individuals obsessively search the internet for health information consequently increasing health anxiety followed by misinterpretation of health symptoms. The instability of emerging adulthood makes individuals vulnerable to the negative consequences of searching for health information online. Cyberchondria is defined as an increased level of health concern or distress linked to recurrent or excessive Online Health Research (OHR) (Starcevic, 2017). Additionally, it has been defined as a 'multidimensional construct' that incorporates 'an element of compulsiveness and negative emotional states or distress associated with Online Health Research' as well as the interruption or disregard of other activities as a result (McElroy & Shevlin, 2014; Starcevic et al., 2021). White and Horvitz (2009) defined cyberchondria as 'the unfounded escalation of concerns about common symptomatology, based on the review of search results and literature on the web'. Repeated and compulsive online searches for health information are a hallmark of cyberchondria, which heightens health anxiety and distress (Infanti et al., 2023). Furthermore, not all internet sources can be trusted, and it can be difficult to separate factual information from inaccurate

DOI: 10.4324/9781003517313-7

or misleading content, which could lead to poor health decisions (Starcevic et al., 2021). Cyberchondria is comprised of four fundamental dimensions which include using the internet excessively to search health-related information, experiencing high levels of stress and anxiety as a result of the information gathered, observing compulsive behaviours and the way that they affect day-to-day activities, and wanting to feel safe (Köse & Murat, 2021). Symptoms of obsessive–compulsive disorder include persistent, recurring thoughts, and behaviours. The definition and classification of cyberchondria are complicated because they incorporate these illnesses' components. It results from excessive searches for health information online (McElroy & Shevlin, 2014). Excessive use of the internet for health-related objectives raises anxiety levels and encourages unwarranted health concerns. In response, McElroy and Shevlin (2014) created the multidimensional Cyberchondria Severity Scale (CSS), a tool for assessing cyberchondria. Cyberchondria is not formally recognised in major diagnostic manuals, such as the Diagnostic and Statistical Manual of Mental Disorders, Fifth Edition (DSM-5), or the International Classification of Diseases 11th Revision (ICD-11), despite its enormous impact on mental health. The lack of it suggests that discussions and investigations on its traits, origins, and diagnostic techniques are still ongoing. According to earlier research, cyberchondria got worse during the COVID-19 pandemic, resulting in reduced comfort-seeking from internet searches but an increase in anxiety and compulsive behaviours (Infanti et al., 2023). Infanti et al. (2023) highlighted the pandemic's consequences on mental health and compulsive online health searches by finding that COVID-19–related health anxiety was a major predictor of cyberchondria.

COVID-19: Fuel to Cyberchondria

Through several interrelated circumstances, the COVID-19 pandemic has contributed to a rise in cyberchondria. Starcevic et al. (2021) model of cyberchondria during the COVID-19 pandemic describes how different factors contribute to the emergence and persistence of cyberchondria in the context of a global health emergency. The model illustrates how psychological and biological vulnerabilities weaken the ability to cope with uncertainty and heighten the sense of threat (Starcevic et al., 2021). People who see COVID-19 as a threat are more likely to search the internet excessively for information relevant to the virus, which is made worse by the number of unreliable and confusing information available online (Starcevic et al., 2021). This obsessive behaviour, which is motivated by a need for validation, feedback into a vicious cycle of heightened anxiety and discomfort, intensifying the sense of danger and unpredictability and encouraging compulsive searching (Starcevic et al., 2021). Several people were terrified and unsure about the virus which made them continually search the internet for information about the symptoms of infection, modes of transmission, and ways to prevent it. This never-ending quest for health information has the potential to create brand-new COVID-19-related anxieties. To contain the spread complete lockdowns and social distancing measures were implemented which resulted in a decrease in physical interactions with healthcare professionals, prompting individuals to rely heavily on the internet for health-related information. This shift towards online sources, while providing some benefits, also led to an overconsumption of information and the proliferation of misinformation related to COVID-19, contributing to heightened levels of anxiety among the searchers. The evolving nature of the COVID-19 virus, coupled with the lack of clear and credible information, created a sense of uncertainty that fuelled compulsive behaviours such as constant monitoring of updates and excessive online searches for reassurance. The combination of increased anxiety, limited access to traditional healthcare services, and the constant barrage of pandemic-related news further exacerbated individuals' health concerns and led to a phenomenon known as cyberchondria. The continuous exposure to COVID-19 news and statistics through various media channels played a significant role in perpetuating health-related fears and maintaining a heightened state of vigilance. Thus, in the aftermath of the COVID-19 pandemic, cyberchondria has emerged as a pressing issue, shaped by persistent health-related anxieties, the vast availability of online information, the continued reliance on telehealth services, and the influential impact of both traditional and social media. The pandemic has indelibly altered public awareness regarding health and illness, resulting in heightened vigilance and ongoing anxiety about personal wellbeing, which drives individuals to seek information on the internet. Concerns surrounding new variants, long-COVID, and other potential health threats perpetuated this cycle of cyberchondria. The volume of health information accessible online has expanded significantly; although many reputable sources exist, the internet is also rife with misinformation and sensationalised narratives. This overwhelming influx of information complicated the task of distinguishing between credible and misleading content, thereby exacerbating cyberchondria.

The pandemic also accelerated the integration of telehealth services, which continued to be favoured in the post-COVID period. While telehealth offered convenient healthcare access, it often led individuals to engage in extensive online searches to complement virtual consultations, which potentially increased their anxiety, particularly when information was misinterpreted. Media coverage of health matters played a crucial role in shaping public perceptions and concerns, with social media platforms amplifying both accurate and erroneous health information. The algorithmic nature of these platforms frequently prioritised engaging content, including alarming or sensational posts, which further intensified health-related anxieties.

Internet Addiction

Cyberchondria has been connected to IA, which is characterised by excessive and uncontrollable online involvement (Servidio et al., 2021; Mrayyan et al., 2022). As the internet becomes more widely available, more people are becoming dependent on it, which presents serious problems for productivity, social interaction, and health. IA is frequently found in people who frequently face emotional problems like loneliness, despair, and anxiety and can show up as excessive usage of social media, online gaming, or other activities. The deluge of false or misleading information available on the internet can exacerbate health fears and lead to problematic internet use, which in turn affects self-esteem, eudaimonic wellbeing, and subjective wellbeing (Ivanova, 2013).

Online health information access has benefits as well as drawbacks. Positively, it can empower people by educating them about a range of health issues, their causes, preventative measures, and available therapies. This can lead to proactive health management and well-informed decision-making (Ivanova, 2013; McMullan et al., 2019). Convenience is another benefit; consumers can easily locate information from reliable sources. But, there are also significant disadvantages. Confusion and misinformation can result from the abundance of information that is readily available, which can be daunting and challenging to navigate. The internet can be utilised by people who are already in distress or apprehensive about their health to self-diagnose or find comfort (White & Horvitz, 2009; McMullan et al, 2019). Singh and Brown (2016) explored the reasons why health-anxious students turn to the internet for health information and the subsequent impact of this behaviour. The study revealed that students sought health information out of curiosity, anxiety regarding undiagnosed symptoms, and the desire to find remedies (Singh & Brown, 2016). Although the internet might offer comfort, it frequently breeds doubt and makes people feel more anxious about their health. Research has demonstrated a connection between cyberchondria, online health information searching, and health anxiety (McMullan et al., 2019). This emphasises how critical it is to exercise caution while consuming internet health information since it has the potential to both exacerbate and lessen health issues, which can have an impact on general wellbeing.

Health Anxiety

According to Marcus et al. (2007), a sizable section of the world's population has health anxiety, which is defined as excessive sensitivity and concern about one's health, frequently stemming from speculative worries about prospective ailments. Health anxiety sufferers often misread little bodily sensations as serious medical conditions, which leads them to continue worrying excessively even when there are no symptoms and they are reassured by doctors. While many people utilise the internet to gather health-related information, those with health anxiety are particularly vulnerable to the negative impacts of such searches. Instead of finding reassurance or valuable knowledge, individuals with health anxiety often experience heightened worry, confusion, and stress as a result of their online health information-seeking behaviours (McMullan et al., 2019). As their anxiety escalates, individuals may engage in more online searches to alleviate their fears (Ivanova, 2013). Furthermore, it was discovered that the association between general anxiety and cyberchondria was moderated by COVID-19 anxiety (Ambrosini et al., 2022). Information processing biases can have a major impact on anxiety disorders. Confirmation bias is the deliberate search for data that confirms preconceived notions (Harvey et al., 2004; Muris et al., 2014). Due to this bias, people tend to ignore or reject evidence that contradicts their pre-existing opinions while favouring and remembering information that supports those opinions (Nickerson, 1998; Westerwick et al., 2017; Gupta et al., 2022; Modgil et al., 2024). For instance, someone who is certain of a diet's efficacy would only read favourable evaluations and ignore any negative ones, which would serve to confirm their initial conviction and possibly exacerbate their concern.

When experiencing symptoms that coincide with their fears of a serious illness, people who suffer from health anxiety may turn to the internet to get information (Brown et al., 2020). Their concerns are heightened by this selective search because vague or confusing information is frequently taken to indicate a serious illness. For example, people may mistakenly think they have a rare disease even though it is unlikely if they read about illnesses with symptoms that resemble their own.

The Interplay of Internet Addiction, Cyberchondria, and Health Anxiety

The intricate relationship between IA, cyberchondria, and health anxiety creates a multifaceted and often harmful cycle that impacts mental health and overall well-being. Those with a predisposition to health anxiety tend to excessively worry about their wellbeing, leading them to seek information online to comprehend their symptoms (McMullan et al., 2019). Online search results frequently present worst-case scenarios, which can be distressing and further intensify concerns. The heightened worries then prompt individuals to continue seeking more information in search of reassurance, resulting in a pattern of compulsive internet use that makes it a challenge to regulate their online behaviour (Ivanova, 2013). The constant need for reassurance fosters reliance on internet searches, and the habit of frequent searching becomes reinforced by the temporary relief found in certain search results (Singh & Brown, 2016). Sometimes people usually view 'health' as something more than just sickness or disease, and they use the internet to be independent and active (Harrod, 2011). However, it can be difficult to evaluate the applicability of the large amount of readily available health information available in various websites, which increases the possibility of misinterpretation and catastrophic thinking (Singh & Brown, 2016). The ongoing cycle of searching and exposure to alarming information exacerbates their health anxiety (Infanti et al., 2023), perpetuating the cycle. Consequently, a feedback loop is established where the deterioration of one condition exacerbates the others, creating a self-sustaining cycle that is difficult to break. This cycle ultimately leads to a significant decline in mental health, as individuals find themselves trapped in a cycle of compulsive behaviour and escalating anxiety.

Objective

The purpose of the study was to explore the relationship between cyberchondria, IA, and health anxiety among emerging adults in North-East India especially in the post-COVID-19 era. In addition to this, the present study attempted to see the differences in health anxiety, cyberchondria, and IA regarding marital status.

Further, through this quantitative approach, the predictors of health anxiety were also explored.

Rationale of the Study

Global mental health has been profoundly affected by the COVID-19 epidemic, with an increase in stress, anxiety, and sadness. Lockdowns and social distancing measures have necessitated an increased reliance on the internet for various purposes, including obtaining information, communication, education, entertainment etc. In the post–COVID-19 scenario, this dependence turned into a regular habit, especially among emerging adults who were worried about the pandemic's long-term health effects, for which they instantly searched for any health-related symptoms online before visiting a physician. This shift marked the increasing role of the internet in the health-related decision-making process, as well as the possible implications for patients and healthcare systems. As a result, the risks of cyberchondria and health-related worries have increased among individuals after COVID-19, due to the reliance on the internet for health information, especially for emerging adults who were already more susceptible to mental health problems, about the North-East region of India. To improve mental health outcomes and guide focused therapies, research on the interaction of cyberchondria, IA, and health anxiety in this area is essential. This research is particularly important in light of the developmental stage of emerging adulthood and the impact of the pandemic on mental health and internet usage.

Method

Sample

The study used a cross-sectional research design, which entails gathering data from a population on different variables at one specific point in time. The 371 emerging adults (188 males), aged between 18 and 29 years, residing in North-East India were selected through snowball sampling. The North-East region of India comprises eight states, namely Arunachal Pradesh, Assam, Meghalaya, Mizoram, Manipur, Nagaland, Tripura, and Sikkim. This area, a picturesque landscape, is known for its rich cultural diversity, with a mix of tribal and non-tribal communities making up most of the population.

Inclusion and Exclusion Criteria

Only emerging adults who had a strong understanding of the English language were selected. Those having a history of substance abuse or psychiatric disorders (such as major depressive disorder, bipolar disorder, or schizophrenia)—whether self-reported or formally diagnosed—were excluded. To maintain the integrity of the consent procedure and the study's ethical guidelines, participants who were incapable of giving informed consent because of cognitive impairments or other problems were excluded. This methodology ensured that the research maintained its cultural and geographical relevance. Helsinki declaration and APA guidelines were strictly adhered to.

Tools

Cyberchondria Severity Scale (CSS) (McElroy & Shevlin, 2014)

The CSS containing 12 items is a self-report questionnaire used to gauge the degree of cyberchondria. It assesses the influence on daily life, anxiety connected to health-related internet searches, and their frequency and intensity. A 5-point scale, ranging from 1 (Never) to 5 (Always), is used to rate each item. The stronger severity of cyberchondria is reflected in higher CSS scores, which also indicate higher frequency and intensity of health searches, higher levels of worry connected to health, and a stronger impact on day-to-day functioning. The cyberchondria scale had a Cronbach alpha of 0.855, indicating good internal consistency.

Internet Addiction Test (IAT) (Young, 2009)

IAT is a self-report questionnaire intended to gauge the extent of IA. It has 20 items, every item is ranked from 0 (Not applicable) to 5 (Always) using a 5-point rating scale. Higher IAT scores are indicative of a severe case of IA, with higher levels of obsession, severe withdrawal symptoms, and substantial negative consequences on day-to-day functioning. The IA scale had a Cronbach alpha of 0.912, indicating excellent internal consistency.

Health Anxiety Inventory (HAI) (Salkovskis et al., 2002)

HAI was used to gauge the degree of health anxiety. The 18 items that make up the HAI assess the frequency and severity of health-related concerns, avoidance behaviours, and how these affect day-to-day functioning. Every item has a 4-point rating scale, ranging from 0 to 3, where higher scores indicate severe health anxiety with the symptoms of greater worry, avoidance, and functional impairment. The HAI had a strong internal consistency with a Cronbach alpha of 0.898.

Procedure

Data were collected between January 2023 and April 2023, with the approval of the institutional ethical committee. The necessary permissions from the authors of the respective scales were obtained for their use. The sets of questionnaires consisted of three parts, beginning with informed consent, followed by a demographic data sheet and questionnaires. Detailed instructions containing the purpose and procedures of the study were given to the participants, assuring them of confidentiality. The questionnaires were shared with the participants using various digital platforms such as email, WhatsApp, and Telegram.

Statistical Analysis

SPSS 20.0 was used to analyse the data. The descriptive statistics (mean, SD, percentage) were calculated to summarise the participants' demographic profiles. To assess the relationships between cyberchondria, IA, and health anxiety, the Spearman correlation was used. The Mann–Whitney *U* test was used to compare married and unmarried emerging adults in terms of health anxiety, cyberchondria, and IA. Finally, regression analysis was done to find out the extent to which health anxiety was predicted by IA and cyberchondria.

Results

According to Table 6.1, the participants' mean age was 23.69 years (SD = 5.78 years). The gender distribution was almost equal, with slightly more males (50.7%) than females (49.3%). The majority of the participants consisted of students (67.4%), followed by employed individuals (22.9%) and unemployed individuals (9.7%). Out of the total participants, only 10.8% were married.

The results indicated a positive and significant correlation between IA and cyberchondria ($\rho = 0.480$, $p < 0.01$) (Table 6.2), suggesting that individuals with cyberchondria tend to exhibit high levels of IA. Furthermore, a positive and

Table 6.1 Demographic profile of the participants ($N = 371$)

	Mean	*SD*	
Age	23.69	5.78	
		Frequency	*Per cent*
Gender	Male	188	50.7
	Female	183	49.3
		Frequency	*Per cent*
Occupational status	Student	250	67.4
	Employed	85	22.9
	Unemployed	36	9.7
		Frequency	*Per cent*
Marital status	Married	40	10.8
	Unmarried	331	89.2

Table 6.2 Correlation between internet addiction, cyberchondria, and health anxiety ($N = 371$)

		Internet addiction	*Cyberchondria*	*Health anxiety*
Spearman's rho	Internet addiction	1	*	
	Cyberchondria	.480**	1	**
	Health anxiety	.436**	.335**	1

** Correlation is significant at the 0.01 level (2-tailed).

Table 6.3 Group differences in health anxiety, cyberchondria, and internet addiction based on marital status ($N = 371$) (Married 40)

	Mean rank	*Mann–Whitney U*	*Z*	*Asymp. Sig. (2-tailed)*
Health anxiety	203.98	5901.000	-1.123	0.261
	183.83			
Cyberchondria	226.48	5001.000	-2.530	0.011
	181.11			
Internet addiction	187.38	6565.000	-0.086	0.932
	185.83			

significant correlation was found between IA and health anxiety ($\rho = 0.436$, $p < 0.01$), indicating that individuals with higher IA levels also tend to experience elevated levels of health anxiety. Additionally, a positive and significant correlation was observed between cyberchondria and health anxiety ($\rho = 0.335$, $p < 0.01$), highlighting the association between higher cyberchondria levels and increased health anxiety. Overall, all correlation coefficients were significant emphasising the significant interrelationships between IA, cyberchondria, and health anxiety.

Table 6.3 shows the group difference in health anxiety, cyberchondria, and IA based on marital status. It is observed that the mean rank for health anxiety was higher among married individuals (203.98) in comparison to unmarried individuals (183.83), although this disparity was not deemed statistically significant ($p = 0.261$), indicating that marital status does not have a significant impact on health anxiety levels within this particular group. Conversely, the mean rank for cyberchondria was notably higher for married individuals (226.48) compared to unmarried individuals (181.11), with a statistically significant difference ($p = 0.011$), suggesting that married individuals exhibited higher levels of cyberchondria in this sample. Furthermore, the mean rank for IA was marginally higher for married individuals (187.38) than unmarried individuals (185.83), yet this discrepancy was not statistically significant ($p = 0.932$). Therefore, based on the findings, it can be concluded that there were no significant differences in IA and health anxiety between married and unmarried individuals, whereas cyberchondria differed significantly between married and unmarried individuals.

Table 6.4 illustrates the proportion of variance in the dependent variable, health anxiety, that can be accounted for by the independent variables, IA, and cyberchondria. The impact of IA on health anxiety (Beta = 0.346) was found to be stronger than cyberchondria (Beta = 0.195) (Table 6.4c). Specifically, 22.8% of the variance in health anxiety was attributed to these two factors (IA and cyberchondria) (Table 6.4a). The finding suggested that the model was statistically significant, $p < 0.01$ (Table 6.4b), which indicated that IA and cyberchondria were significant predictors of health anxiety; however, it also implied that there were 77.2% of the variability in health anxiety remains unexplained by IA and cyberchondria.

Table 6.4 Predictors of health anxiety in emerging adults

Table 6.4 (a) Model summary

Model	*R*	*R Square*	*Adjusted R square*	*Std. Error of the estimate*
1	0.478[a]	0.228	0.224	8.420

[a] Predictors: (Constant), internet addiction, cyberchondria.

Table 6.4 (b) ANOVA[a]

Model	*Sum of squares*	*df*	*Mean square*	*F*	*Sig.*	
1	Regression	7712.200	2	3856.100	54.380	0.000[b]
	Residual	26095.110	368	70.911		
	Total	33807.310	370			

[a] Dependent variable: Health anxiety.
[b] Predictors: (Constant), internet addiction, cyberchondria.

Table 6.4 (c) Coefficients

Model		*Unstandardised coefficients*		*Standardised coefficients*	*t*	*Sig.*
		B	*Std. Error*	*Beta*		
1	Constant	2.434	1.732		1.405	0.161
	Cyberchondria	0.230	0.063	0.195	3.645	0.000
	Internet addiction	0.201	0.031	0.346	6.457	0.000

[a] Dependent variable: Health anxiety.

Discussion

Internet users make considerable use of online health resources because the internet is a vital source of health information nowadays (Te Poel et al., 2016; Dagar et al., 2019; Polat et al., 2022). The present study revealed a strong correlation between IA and cyberchondria suggesting that emerging adults from North-East India were more likely to be addicted to the internet, which can worsen health anxiety and lead to excessive online searches for health information. In line with the present findings, previous research has also observed a significant connection between IA and health anxiety (Polat et al., 2022; Mrayyan et al., 2022). This research highlighted the risks of excessive internet browsing for mental health. Consistent with our findings, prior research indicated a strong relationship between smartphone addiction and frequent searches for online health-related information during the COVID-19 pandemic (Köse & Murat, 2021). Dong et al. (2020) noted in their observations that people were frequently using their phones and the internet excessively to cope with the stress and uncertainty brought on by the pandemic. This is consistent with our research, which discovered that increased usage of the internet for health-related information was associated with IA. This association makes sense when it is considered how people's fears and anxieties can get worse when they look for health information repeatedly (Starcevic, 2017; Avçin & Can, 2022).

A strong positive correlation between cyberchondria and health anxiety was observed in the present study. It indicated that people who experienced higher levels of cyberchondria also perceived higher levels of health anxiety because people with cyberchondria engage in excessive and recurrent online searches for health information. Their behaviour exhibited a form of compulsive internet use that is indicative of IA. When internet addicts search for health-related information online, they frequently come across scary or dubious content, which exacerbates their worry. In a similar vein, Ivanova (2013) also found noteworthy connections between IA and health anxiety triggered by searching health information online and the persistence and intensification of concerns. Thus, there seems to be a connection between excessive internet use, searches for health information online, and ensuing worries about one's health (Ivanova, 2013). Cyberchondria sufferers get momentary relief from ostensibly explanatory material, which reinforces their behaviour. This pattern is comparable to other forms of IA in which instant reward increases the urge to use the internet. Since there is already a well-established connection between IA and health anxiety, treating the former may help to reduce the latter. Online health information that is sensationalised or inconsistent can make people feel more anxious about their health. Singh and Brown (2016) discovered that although those with high levels of health anxiety spent more time and conducted more searches online, their anxiety did not go down. Since excessive online health searches frequently amplify worry and health concerns, higher degrees of cyberchondria are correlated with higher levels of health anxiety (Ivanova, 2013; Infanti et al., 2023). When looking for health information online, people are more likely to come across disturbing content, which makes them feel more anxious about their health. Exaggerating these discoveries and fretting over the repercussions, cyberchondriacs often track actual changes in their bodies (Polat et al., 2022) and thus anxiety is increased by this behaviour (Fergus & Spada, 2017; Gül et al., 2016). According to a meta-analysis published in 2019, individuals who engage in cyberchondria behaviours report feeling more anxious about their health (McMullan et al., 2019). Also, the present findings showed that health anxiety was strongly predicted by IA and cyberchondria, indicating that internet addicts spend a lot of time online, where they come across conflicting or unpleasant health information, which in turn makes them more anxious about their health. The findings show that marital status has a major impact on cyberchondria, but not health anxiety or IA. The necessity to keep an eye on possible health issues affecting family members may contribute to a higher incidence of cyberchondria among married individuals. Compulsive searches for health information might result from anxiety over the health of loved ones, as people look for comfort in the knowledge that their loved ones are doing well.

Limitations

This study focused on emerging adults, hence its findings could not be applied to other populations. Additionally, the study's exclusive focus on North-East India may limit the findings' applicability to areas with different socio-economic and cultural circumstances.

Suggestions

Researchers should conduct investigations which ought to investigate the supplementary factors that contribute to health anxiety to accommodate greater variation and demonstrate causal connections via longitudinal studies. The significant variability in health anxiety remains unexplained by IA and cyberchondria due to the presence of additional factors that were not included in the present study. These unaccounted factors may include personal health history, genetic predisposition, anxiety levels, social support, and other environmental or psychological variables. Therefore, it is important to consider these additional factors in future research to gain a more comprehensive understanding of the determinants of health anxiety.

Conclusion

Mental health concerns have gained attention because of the increase in digital communication and availability of online health information, especially after the COVID-19 pandemic. The study finds a substantial correlation between cyberchondria, online addiction, and health anxiety, demonstrating that persons with higher levels of cyberchondria also have higher levels of IA and health worry. These results highlight the intricate interactions between these illnesses and suggest that frequent health searches and excessive internet use may exacerbate health issues. Reducing health anxiety and enhancing mental wellbeing requires addressing IA and promoting safe online conduct.

Acknowledgements

We extend our heartfelt gratitude to all who support the development of this chapter, with special thanks to our mentors and colleagues for their invaluable feedback and to the editor for his guidance and patience throughout the process.

Conflict of Interest

Nil.

References

Ambrosini, F., Truzoli, R., Vismara, M., Vitella, D., & Biolcati, R. (2022). The effect of cyberchondria on anxiety, depression and quality of life during COVID-19: The mediational role of obsessive-compulsive symptoms and Internet addiction. *Heliyon, 8*(5), 1–9.

Arnett, J. J. (2000). Emerging adulthood: A theory of development from the late teens through the twenties. *American Psychologist, 55*(5), 469–480.

Arnett, J. J., Žukauskienė, R., & Sugimura, K. (2014). The new life stage of emerging adulthood at ages 18–29 years: Implications for mental health. *The Lancet Psychiatry, 1*(7), 569–576.

Avçin, E., & Can, Ş. (2022). The relationship between the stress experienced by parents and cyberchondria during the pandemic process. *Library Hi Tech, 40*(2), 548–568.

Brown, R. J., Skelly, N., & Chew-Graham, C. A. (2020). Online health research and health anxiety: A systematic review and conceptual integration. *Clinical Psychology: Science and Practice, 27*(2), 20.

Dagar, D., Kakodkar, P., & Shetiya, S. H. (2019). Evaluating the cyberchondria construct among computer engineering students in Pune (India) using Cyberchondria Severity Scale (CSS-15). *Indian Journal of Occupational and Environmental Medicine, 23*(3), 117–120.

Dong, H., Yang, F., Lu, X., & Hao, W. (2020). Internet addiction and related psychological factors among children and adolescents in China during the coronavirus disease 2019 (COVID-19) epidemic. *Frontiers in Psychiatry, 11*, 751. https://doi.org/10.3389/fpsyt.2020.00751

Fergus, T. A., & Spada, M. M. (2017). Cyberchondria: Examining relations with problematic internet use and metacognitive beliefs. *Clinical Psychology & Psychotherapy, 24*(6), 1322–1330. https://doi.org/10.1002/cpp.2086

Gül, A. İ., Özdemir, T., & Börekçi, E. (2016). Health anxiety levels in patients admitted to internal medicine outpatient clinic for several times. *Journal of Clinical and Analytical Medicine, 7*(4), 437–439. https://doi.org/10.4328/JCAM.3990

Gupta, M., Parra, C. M., & Dennehy, D. (2022). Questioning racial and gender bias in AI-based recommendations: Do espoused national cultural values matter? *Information Systems Frontiers, 24*(5), 1465–1481. https://doi.org/10.1007/s10796-021-10190-5

Harrod, M. (2011). "I have to keep going": Why some older adults are using the internet for health information. *Ageing International, 36*(3), 283–294. https://doi.org/10.1007/s12126-011-9113-2

Harvey, A. G., Watkins, E., & Mansell, W. (2004). *Cognitive Behavioural Processes across Psychological Disorders: A Transdiagnostic Approach to Research and Treatment.* Oxford University Press.

Infanti, A., Starcevic, V., Schimmenti, A., Khazaal, Y., Karila, L., Giardina, A., & Billieux, J. (2023). Predictors of cyberchondria during the COVID-19 pandemic: Cross-sectional study using supervised machine learning. *JMIR Formative Research, 7*(1), e42206. https://doi.org/10.2196/42206

Ivanova, E. (2013). Internet addiction and cyberchondria: Their relationship with well-being. *The Journal of Education, Culture, and Society, 4*(1), 57–70. https://doi.org/10.15503/jecs20131.57.70

Köse, S., & Murat, M. (2021). Examination of the relationship between smartphone addiction and cyberchondria in adolescents. *Archives of Psychiatric Nursing, 35*(6), 563–570. https://doi.org/10.1016/j.apnu.2021.08.015

Marcus, D. K., Gurley, J. R., Marchi, M. M., & Bauer, C. (2007). Cognitive and perceptual variables in hypochondriasis and health anxiety: A systematic review. *Clinical Psychology Review, 27*(2), 127–139. https://doi.org/10.1016/j.cpr.2006.09.003

McElroy, E., & Shevlin, M. (2014). The development and initial validation of the cyberchondria severity scale (CSS). *Journal of Anxiety Disorders, 28*(2), 259–265. https://doi.org/10.1016/j.janxdis.2013.12.007

McMullan, R. D., Berle, D., Arnáez, S., & Starcevic, V. (2019). The relationships between health anxiety, online health information seeking, and cyberchondria: Systematic review and meta-analysis. *Journal of Affective Disorders, 245*, 270–278. https://doi.org/10.1016/j.jad.2018.11.037

Modgil, S., Singh, R. K., Gupta, S., & Dennehy, D. (2024). A confirmation bias view on social media induced polarization during COVID-19. *Information Systems Frontiers, 26*(2), 417–441. https://doi.org/10.1007/s10796-022-10290-7

Mrayyan, M. T., Al-Rawashdeh, S., Khait, A. A., & Rababa, M. (2022). Differences in cyberchondria, internet addiction, anxiety sensitivity, health anxiety, and coronavirus anxiety among students: A web-based comparative survey. *Electronic Journal of General Medicine, 19*(3), em366. https://doi.org/10.29333/ejgm/11922

Muris, P., Debipersad, S., & Mayer, B. (2014). Searching for danger: On the link between worry and threat-related confirmation bias in children. *Journal of Child and Family Studies, 23*, 604–609. https://doi.org/10.1007/s10826-013-9721-5

Nickerson, R. S. (1998). Confirmation bias: A ubiquitous phenomenon in many guises. *Review of General Psychology, 2*(2), 175–220. https://doi.org/10.1037/1089-2680.2.2.175

Polat, F., Delibaş, L., & Bilir, İ. (2022). Investigating the relationship between cyberchondria level and perceived stress in young adults. *Turkish Journal of Science and Health, 3*(3), 176–184. https://doi.org/10.51972/tfsd.1114582

Salkovskis, P. M., Rimes, K. A., Warwick, H. M., & Clark, D. (2002). The Health Anxiety Inventory: Development and validation of scales for the measurement of health anxiety and hypochondriasis. *Psychological Medicine, 32*(5), 843–853. https://doi.org/10.1017/S0033291702005822

Servidio, R., Bartolo, M. G., Palermiti, A. L., & Costabile, A. (2021). Fear of COVID-19, depression, anxiety, and their association with internet addiction disorder in a sample of Italian students. *Journal of Affective Disorders Reports, 4*, 100097. https://doi.org/10.1016/j.jadr.2021.100097

Singh, K., & Brown, R. J. (2016). From headache to tumour: An examination of health anxiety, health-related internet use and 'query escalation'. *Journal of Health Psychology, 21*(9), 2008–2020. https://doi.org/10.1177/1359105315578312

Singh, K., Fox, J. R., & Brown, R. J. (2016). Health anxiety and Internet use: A thematic analysis. *Cyberpsychology: Journal of Psychosocial Research on Cyberspace, 10*(2), Article 2. https://doi.org/10.5817/CP2016-2-5

Starcevic, V. (2017). Cyberchondria: Challenges of problematic online searches for health-related information. *Psychotherapy and Psychosomatics, 86*(3), 129–133. https://doi.org/10.1159/000465525

Starcevic, V., Schimmenti, A., Billieux, J., & Berle, D. (2021). Cyberchondria in the time of the COVID-19 pandemic. *Human Behaviour and Emerging Technologies, 3*(1), 53–62. https://doi.org/10.1002/hbe2.233

Te Poel, F., Baumgartner, S. E., Hartmann, T., & Tanis, M. (2016). The curious case of cyberchondria: A longitudinal study on the reciprocal relationship between health anxiety and online health information seeking. *Journal of Anxiety Disorders, 43*, 32–40. https://doi.org/10.1016/j.janxdis.2016.07.009

Westerwick, A., Johnson, B. K., & Knobloch-Westerwick, S. (2017). Confirmation biases in selective exposure to political online information: Source bias vs. content bias. *Communication Monographs, 84*(3), 343–364. https://doi.org/10.1080/03637751.2016.1272761

White, R. W., & Horvitz, E. (2009). Cyberchondria: Studies of the escalation of medical concerns in web search. *ACM Transactions on Information Systems (TOIS), 27*(4), Article 23. https://doi.org/10.1145/1629096.1629101

Young, K. S. (2009). *Internet Addiction Test*. Center for Online Addictions. www.netaddiction.com

7 Unveiling the Experiences of Women Domestic Workers in India Amid and Beyond the COVID-19 Pandemic

A Narrative Review

Swathy Sathyapal

Introduction

The informal sector is a significant part of the employment landscape in India. The urban employment sector predominantly comprises informal employment, accounting for up to 90% of the workforce, as reported by the International Labour Organization (ILO, 2018), of which domestic workers form a crucial yet underreported group. In a recent survey by the Ministry of Labour and Employment (2023), about 28.1 million domestic and household workers have been documented across India. However, organisations like the ILO (2010) and the National Domestic Workers Movement (n.d) report that unofficial estimates indicate upward of 50 million workers, highlighting the glaring lack of official data on this vulnerable population. The majority of these workers are women, generally earning below minimum wages, and less than their male counterparts (Raveendran & Vanek, 2020). Despite their considerable numbers and significant contributions, they are often socially and legally overlooked as a group in India, without a solid legislative framework to protect their rights.

The Coronavirus disease 2019 (COVID-19) pandemic exacerbated the existing vulnerabilities of these women domestic workers (WDWs), highlighting the severe injustices, inequities, and loss of dignity they face (Chen, 2020). The World Health Organization (WHO, 2020) noted that informal workers, particularly women, faced increased risks due to minimal social protection and poor access to healthcare. In India, these workers experienced significant job insecurity and wage losses amounting to ₹635.53 billion during the pandemic (Estupinan & Sharma, 2020). Additionally, the extended lockdown and mobility restrictions hindered their ability to resume work consequently slowing their financial recovery (Ismail & Ogando, 2023).

Further, research shows that the pandemic has had a gendered impact globally and in India, disproportionately affecting women more than men, in terms of employment and income, healthcare risks, heightened domestic stress and care burdens, and domestic violence, among others (Abraham et al., 2022; Deshpande, 2020). This trend is especially pronounced among India's WDWs who lack formal employment benefits and social protection. Gender, caste, class, and informal work status have combined to uniquely challenge and marginalise

DOI: 10.4324/9781003517313-8

these women (Singh & Kaur, 2022). Early assessments painted a bleak picture for WDWs, revealing insufficient government support in ensuring income continuity, social security, or food security, along with heavier unpaid domestic work (Dasgupta & Mitra, 2020). However, the government had announced some support measures such as relief packages for some labourers and industries, and direct cash transfers for many poor and vulnerable women, though the efficiency and scale of the relief measures have been pointed out to be inadequate (Kujur & Goswami, 2020).

Due to the limited literature on this group, most researchers adopt a primarily qualitative method, offering some insights into different aspects of this population. However, there is a dearth of studies using a quantitative approach and a need for a synthesised overview of their experiences brought on by the pandemic to provide a comprehensive understanding of their myriad challenges and identify the personal and structural factors that have shaped their experiences during this tumultuous period. Furthermore, this can serve to identify gaps and issues in existing policies and support measures. This can offer the groundwork to advocate for more inclusive and effective measures to safeguard the wellbeing and rights of WDWs in the evolving post-pandemic landscape.

Objectives

The objective of this study was to provide a comprehensive review of the existing literature on the experiences and challenges faced by WDWs during and after the COVID-19 pandemic, present key findings, and identify potential ways forward.

Method

This narrative review identified relevant literature between March 2020 and April 2024 through thorough searches for original and peer-reviewed articles across electronic databases including PubMed, Scopus, and PsycINFO using specific search terms (Table 7.1). Additional searches were conducted through Google Scholar along with manual searches of journal articles and bibliographies to further identify relevant studies. Research articles and materials published online focusing on Indian women engaged in paid domestic work, highlighting experiences during or after the COVID-19 pandemic, and addressing mental, emotional, or behavioural challenges were included. Studies were excluded if they did not meet the study objectives, were not written in English, were not available in full text or were considered to be grey literature. The titles and abstracts of original articles were screened and selected based on their fit with the inclusion criteria. A detailed review of the eight primary studies that shaped the major themes has been given in Table 7.2. Due to the limited literature and the predominant use of qualitative methods in the selected studies, a narrative review method was chosen instead of a systematic review or a meta-analysis.

Table 7.1 List of databases, search terms utilised, and criteria for inclusion of studies

Databases (Between March 2020 and April 2024)	*List of search terms*	*Selection criteria*
PubMed Scopus PsycINFO	'female domestic workers', OR 'women domestic workers' OR 'domestic workers' AND 'COVID-19' OR 'pandemic' AND 'impact' OR 'effect' OR 'experience' AND 'India'	**Inclusion criteria:** 1. Primary research studies investigating: a. experiences of Indian women engaged in domestic work. b. during or after the COVID-19 pandemic. c. address mental, emotional, or behavioural challenges. 2. Published in peer-reviewed journals in the English language. **Exclusion criteria:** 1. Published in editorials, commentaries, discussion papers, or conference abstracts. 2. Gray literature. 3. Not published in English language.

Findings

Pre-existing Vulnerabilities

WDWs in India, which mainly include mostly illiterate or minimally educated migrant women, have historically faced significant vulnerabilities that impacted their lives and livelihoods in the urban employment sector (Raveendran & Vanek, 2020).

The sector is characterised by low wages and the absence of formal contracts, leaving many workers vulnerable to unpaid overtime, occupational health issues, and exploitative working conditions that include mental, physical, and sexual violence, human rights violations, and a significant lack of legal or organisational support or representation (Bhattacharya et al., 2016; Neetha, 2009). Further, the lack of access to education and training significantly hinders their upward mobility (Sahoo, 2023). Given their exclusion from organisational benefits like pensions or bonuses, such conditions also restrict their ability to attain financial security to meet basic needs or to save for emergencies and plan for retirement (Ugargol & Parvathy, 2022).

In a mixed-method study on domestic workers in Mysore, Daraei and Mohajery (2013) found that employers saw their domestic workers as 'servants' more than as employees and felt no guilt in exploiting them. Within their workplace, the employer–employee dynamic in this sector is fraught with inequalities and

Table 7.2 Studies reviewed related to the experiences of WDWs during and after the pandemic

S. No	*Author*	*Title of study*	*Publisher*	*Study design*	*Location*	*Sample*	*Main findings*
1	Sumalatha et al. (2021)	Impact of Covid-19 on Informal Sector: A Study of Women Domestic Workers in India	SAGE Journals	Mixed methods including quantitative and qualitative data collected over telephonic conversations	Delhi, Mumbai and Kochi	*N*=260 DWs (age range 18–65 years) selected by random samplingfor the survey, *N*=12 DWs selected by purposive sampling for the telephonic interviews.	- Widespread job loss and wage losses were reported, although there was some employer support. - The short-term impacts on participants and their families included rent difficulties, restricted food, lack of food variety, increased workload, and increased domestic violence, whereas long-term impacts were increased debts, forced asset sales, job and financial insecurity, and marital stress. - Though government support was received to an extent, the participants reported that it was not enough to meet their expenditures through the pandemic.

2	Banerjee & Wilks (2022)	Work in pandemic times: Exploring precarious continuities in paid domestic work in India	Wiley	Qualitative interview method	Delhi and Kolkata	N=15 WDWs (age range=20–55 years), and representatives from an NGO and a labour rights organisation selected by purposive sampling	- WDWs experienced increased job and housing insecurity along with increased control and surveillance at home. - Decreased bargaining power and stigmatised avoidance behaviours even when returning to work was reported. - Paid domestic work was found to be shaped by and reproduce existing gender, class, and caste divides.
3	Bhat et al. (2022)	Fear, discrimination, and healthcare access during the COVID-19 pandemic: Exploring women domestic workers' lives in India	Routledge	Mixed methods including quantitative survey and qualitative interviews	Kochi, Delhi, and Mumbai	N=150 WDWs (age range= 18–62 years) in the quantitative study, selected by simple random sampling. N=40 in the qualitative study.	- WDWs had increased workloads, limited healthcare access, increased domestic violence, and faced stigma and discrimination which were also gendered in nature. - Sleeplessness, a trust deficit, and experiences of a loss of dignity were reported.

(Continued)

Table 7.2 (Continued)

S. No	*Author*	*Title of study*	*Publisher*	*Study design*	*Location*	*Sample*	*Main findings*
4	Gupta et al. (2022)	How COVID-19 Affected the Work Prospects and Healthcare-Seeking of Women Domestic Workers in Kolkata City, India? A Longitudinal Study	Wolters Kluwer	Longitudinal analysis from early 2020 and mid-2020	Slums of Kalikapur locality of Kolkata city, West Bengal	*N*=292 WDWs (aged up to 65 years), selected by random sampling method	- The majority of the participants lost jobs by mid-2020 and had decreased work hours. Concurrently, there were significant monthly pay reductions and a fall in mean family income levels. - By mid-2020, healthcare seeking was significantly negatively impacted through decreased visits to health practitioners, increased over-the-counter medicine use, and ignoring of symptoms.
5	Singh & Kaur (2022)	The COVID-19 pandemic: Narratives of informal women workers in Indian Punjab	Wiley	Qualitative research following Intersectionality analysis framework	Mohali district, Punjab	*N*=34 informal workers (mean age=31.5 years) of which six were WDWs, selected by maximum variation purposive sampling	- There was poverty-related stresses and livelihood challenges, heightened food insecurity, restrictions on mobility, reproductive health issues along with disruption of routine health services, and social ostracism

6	Mohan et al. (2022)	Gauging the impact of a pandemic on the lives and livelihoods of female domestic worker across Indian cities	Universidad Tecnica de Manabi, and ScienceScholar Institution	Survey	Pune, Lucknow, Jhansi, Katni and Bhopal	N=250 WDWs (mean age= 40 years), selected by random sampling	- As incomes fell, consumption patterns shifted, leading to a decline in nutrient-rich foods, depletion of personal savings, increased borrowing from formal and informal sources, and greater reliance on government aid, though insufficient. - There were significant city-level differences, with Jhansi having the highest job loss, followed by Lucknow, Katni, Bhopal, and Pune.
7	Bhattacharjee & Sharma (2023)	A gendered approach to examining pandemic-induced livelihood crisis in the informal sector: The case of female domestic workers in Titwala	CRC Press	Qualitative survey method	Titwala, an extended suburb of Mumbai, Maharashtra	N=38 WDWs (Ages unspecified), selected by random sampling	- WDWs experienced income loss, reduced bargaining power, and increased debts even after the lockdown ended. - Increased domestic workload and stigma at workplace because of being considered unclean were reported. - Children's educations were disrupted exacerbating existing insecurities

(*Continued*)

Table 7.2 (Continued)

S. No	*Author*	*Title of study*	*Publisher*	*Study design*	*Location*	*Sample*	*Main findings*
8	Kumar and Baliyan (2023)	The Impact of the COVID-19 Pandemic on Female Domestic Workers in an Urban Setting	Springer	Primary survey using interviews and focus group discussions	Lucknow city	*N*=72 WDWs (age range= 15 and above 60)	- WDWs faced significant emotional and social consequences due to the pandemic, including financial distress, shortage of food and rations, increased stress and health problems, dual burden of work at home and outside, increased domestic violence, and increased demands at home. - The effects were even more heightened during the second wave than the first.

exploitation with domestic workers often subjected to mistrust and exploitation within the very homes they maintain (Dickey, 2000). Perhaps this also stems from the intersection of historically maintained societal hierarchies of class, caste, and gender, which stigmatises and dehumanises those from lower socio-economic classes and castes as 'others' and not deserving of equal rights (Seedat-Khan et al., 2014). The boundary lines of caste also dictate the types of work allocated to domestic workers, based on notions of purity and pollution that pervade Indian society (Raval & Nizami, 2024).

The challenges extend into the domestic sphere, where the work–life balance becomes a contentious issue, often leading to familial disputes exacerbated by factors such as alcoholism within the household (Khillare & Sonawane, 2016). These issues are also compounded by health problems, particularly musculoskeletal disorders, respiratory illnesses, and non-fatal injuries, which have higher rates of prevalence among WDWs, underscoring the occupational hazards they face that affect all spheres of their life (Alex et al., 2022).

Despite the crucial role WDWs play, the lack of recognition, coupled with the absence of formal contracts and legislative protection, severely undermines their negotiating power and leaves them disempowered (Bhattacharya et al., 2016; Sahni & Junnarkar, 2019). Chadha (2020) describes the lack of official data on the number and profile of the workers and the incoherent legal and policy actions that exclude them from the protective umbrella of labour laws. Additionally, it is difficult for the WDWs to organise into trade unions or other formal institutions which are largely male-dominated, also due to the lack of a common workplace (Sahni & Junnarkar, 2019), though some formal and informal groups do exist that have significantly made strides in empowering and advocating for their rights (Parpiani, 2021). However, these groups face difficulties in gaining formal recognition, and funds, and limitations in reaching the workers (Singh & Kaur, 2022).

In sum, this section highlighted the pre-existing socio-economic plight of Indian WDWs that work to reduce their bargaining power, leaving them vulnerable to exploitation, stigmatisation, and systemic neglect (Bhattacharjee & Goswami, 2020).

COVID-19 Pandemic and WDWs

Impact of the Pandemic on Employment and Income

As the COVID-19 pandemic spread and the lockdown was initiated, the immediate effect on WDWs was abrupt and widespread job loss and wage cuts (Anand, 2021). This translated into significantly decreased consumption, expenditure, and access to medical facilities throughout the pandemic, as noted by Mohan et al. (2022), in their study on 250 WDWs from five Indian cities including Pune, Lucknow, Jhansi, Katni, and Bhopal. Many women were forced to accept lower-paying jobs as they struggled to meet basic expenses, resorting to increased borrowings, leading to dwindling savings and mounting debts. Job loss of other earning family members also increased the burden on these women to make ends meet as they became the sole breadwinners for their families (Gupta et al., 2022). Intergenerational ripple effects of the wage cuts were seen in Bhattacharjee and Sharma's (2023) study on WDWs in Titwala, an extended residential suburb of Mumbai, through the discontinuation of children's education due to lack of access to smartphones and online technologies during tight financial times where basic survival needs took precedence over affording data packs.

Through a comprehensive study including WDWs, NGO practitioners, and labour rights activists in Delhi and Kolkata, Banerjee and Wilks (2022) noted that renegotiations over jobs and wages, coupled with the lack of formal or legal job contracts, led to increased feelings of insecurity and helplessness among WDWs.

Ghatak and Sarkar (2022) found a deterioration in employment and employer–employee relationships for WDWs in Ahmedabad and Kolkata during the pandemic. For WDWs, the replaceability of their labour became starkly evident as employers opted for cheaper labour or took on household chores themselves, further casting doubt on their post-pandemic job security (Banerjee & Wilks, 2022). Thus, despite severe mobility restrictions during strict and repeated lockdowns, some workers continued to work out of necessity, underlining the precarious continuities that shape their livelihoods. These groups were concerned about eviction too, which was particularly acute among women who did not own their homes, especially migrant workers.

Moreover, the gendered effect was highlighted by Bhat et al. (2022) in their study on 150 WDWs from three Indian metropolitan cities in the South, North, and West parts of the country covering Kochi, Delhi, and Mumbai. The participants reported that while WDWs were given wage cuts, men in similar service roles like security guards, did not experience a similar financial setback by the same employers.

The plight of migrant workers, particularly highlighted by media during the pandemic, revealed their dilemma: returning to their hometowns risking travel during a pandemic, or staying in urban centres amid the uncertainty (Jesline et al., 2021; Jha & Lahiri, 2020). Migrant WDWs who stayed often lived in informal settlements or slums, facing challenges due to sudden job loss and movement restrictions (Bhattacharjee & Sharma, 2023). They also faced barriers in accessing pandemic aid and were often even excluded from state relief measures due to difficulties in documentation (Ismail & Ogando, 2023).

However, the effects on WDWs were not entirely uniform throughout India. City-wise disparities emerged during the lockdown, with variations in employment continuity and income levels across different urban centres (Mohan et al., 2022; Sumalatha et al., 2021). However, the reason for the same has not been discussed in most of the literature.

Health, Occupational Risks, and Safety Concerns

The COVID-19 pandemic has not only disrupted economic stability but also, directly and indirectly, impacted the health and wellbeing of WDWs in India, amplifying existing occupational risks and safety concerns. The pandemic saw a significant decline in visits to healthcare practitioners, as reported by Gupta et al. (2022) in a longitudinal study on WDWs residing in Kalikapur, a slum locality of Kolkata City, West Bengal. Concurrently, the authors noted a rising reliance on over-the-counter medications and a concerning trend of ignoring health symptoms, likely driven by economic constraints and fear of exposure to the virus from hospitals. The overall cost of medicines rose, further straining their already limited financial resources (Mohan et al., 2022). Kumar and Baliyan's (2023) study on 72 WDWs from Lucknow reports the increased risk faced by workers due to cramped living spaces and difficulty following hygiene practices and social distancing. As a result, WDWs reported higher levels of anxiety, stress, and disturbed sleep patterns (Sumalatha et al., 2021).

Pre-existing challenges in accessing affordable healthcare were exacerbated, with healthcare services stretched thin and prioritising COVID-19-related treatment (Banerjee & Wilks, 2022). This situation severely affected women's reproductive health, leading to complications such as unwanted pregnancies, miscarriages, and other health issues (Singh & Kaur, 2022), and the discontinuation of treatments for chronic conditions due to non-affordability of medicines and lack of support (Bhat et al., 2022). Thus, many women concealed any potential signs of illnesses at work fearing stigma and the high costs associated with COVID-19 testing and quarantine demanded by employers. Some of the reasons for delays in seeking needed healthcare include heightened domestic burdens (Dey et al., 2022) and misinformation and misconceptions about the disease, like the fear of forceful quarantining and dying alone (Ramani et al., 2022).

Bhat et al.'s (2022) study highlighted some of the inadequacies of the healthcare system, especially for members of marginalised communities, particularly women. The authors noted that the sudden diversion of resources to pandemic responses and increased workloads for health workers impeded their access to relevant information and care. Moreover, the gender-insensitive health communication strategies often left them out of the conversation and unable to advocate for their health needs, failing to provide them with accessible information about the disease, its prevention, and treatment (Pinchoff et al., 2020). Notably, Anusuya et al.'s (2022) study on rural domestic workers from Mizoram, found that despite their fears, many participants obtained their COVID-19 information from the media and had a good understanding of its spread and prevention.

Alongside a health crisis, the pandemic also quickly developed into a hunger and malnutrition crisis through global food insecurity and more individuals being pushed to extreme poverty (Bhargava & Bhargava, 2021). The ability of vulnerable communities, including WDWs, to consume adequate and nutritious food was gravely impacted, with a significant decline in food intake (Mohan et al., 2022; Sumalatha et al., 2021). NGOs and religious organisations like gurdwaras and temples which emerged as the only provision of food for many, too, were often affected by lockdown restrictions (Singh & Kaur, 2022). Although some recovery in income and consumption levels has been noted post-pandemic, indicating a prolonged period of nutritional deficiency and its potential long-term health implications for the WDWs as well as their children (Mohan et al., 2022).

Social Stigma and Isolation

The COVID-19 pandemic exacerbated the combination of social shame, isolation, and economic vulnerability, particularly for WDWs in India who had to navigate the intersections of class, and caste amid a global health crisis. A study by Sumalatha et al. (2021) involving 260 WDWs from three urban cities revealed that more than 57% encountered stigma and discrimination at work, often being humiliated and projected as carriers of the virus during the pandemic. The stigma was not only perpetuated by employers but also by gated communities and resident welfare associations that reinforced negative stereotypes of workers as dirty, fuelling a climate of fear and mistrust. Further, the lack of intervention measures against the stigma from the government was also noted. Aligning with this, Bhat et al. (2022) reported that the overall wellbeing and quality of life decreased for many domestic workers who have reported increased instances of sleeplessness, a significant trust deficit, and experiences of loss of dignity, both at the workplace and while commuting. Reports of verbal abuse by police personnel and derogatory labelling, such as being called greedy for seeking work during a health crisis, underscore the multiple layers of stigma they confronted. Bhat et al.'s (2022) study further underscored the gendered nature of this discrimination, noting that these women travelling for work were often treated as law violators and subjected to abuse, including by police personnel, whereas men's movements were typically justified as necessary for earning a livelihood. In addition, they were also often humiliated and belittled when seeking information about the virus and its prevention measures, reinforcing their marginal status and exacerbating their vulnerability, leaving them ill-equipped to protect themselves and their families from the virus.

According to Banerjee and Wilks (2022), the pandemic has reignited existing caste and class-based prejudices compounded by contemporary notions of 'hygiene' and 'distancing', manifesting in avoidance behaviours and dehumanising and discriminatory practices that label lower-class workers as 'dirty' and disease spreaders. Aligning with existing notions of some communities as 'impure' and 'dirty outsiders' in India (Waghmore & Contractor, 2015), the authors found evidence that domestic workers have faced intense discrimination, resulting in heightened social distancing, harassment, and job losses during the pandemic. Similarly, migrant workers too, were stigmatised and othered during the pandemic, with the sudden lockdowns announced (Choolayil & Putran, 2021). In addition to the hardship of their journeys back home, they carried the weight of added stigma and were often treated without dignity during and after their exodus home (Jha & Lahiri, 2020). Further, women migrant workers have been found to have greater barriers to overall post-COVID-19 recovery than men, with long-term impacts (Allard et al., 2022).

Thus, WDWs have faced significant injustices due to stigma and prejudices during the pandemic, primarily caused by systemic inequalities including lack of social and legal support.

Domestic Stress and Care Burden Amidst the Pandemic

With wages dwindling, extra workloads, healthcare systems inaccessible, and schools closed, the pandemic has significantly amplified the domestic stress and care burden for WDWs in India, intertwining with the country's deep-rooted patriarchal norms, to exacerbate the challenges they face within their households.

Bhat et al. (2022) report widespread feelings of confusion, restlessness, and psychological stress among WDWs. School closures and healthcare system strains increased their caregiving load as the full family presence at home significantly added to their daily responsibilities and domestic chores, as noted by Sumalatha et al. (2021). The constant presence of family members in tightly confined living spaces not only intensified the workload but also caused more family conflicts and privacy issues, severely impacting women's quality of life and reducing their time for rest, recreation, and social interactions. This is also punctuated by decreased food intake, self-care behaviours, and healthcare-seeking among women, primarily due to the exhaustive nature of their responsibilities, which left little to no time for self-care or rest (Gupta et al., 2022). The fear of future lockdowns and a lack of state social security measures have further heightened their distress (Anand, 2021).

The gendered division of housework visibly became apparent during the lockdown as the economic and emotional burden of household management disproportionately fell on the women, experiencing income loss as well as a significant increase in domestic workload (Bhattacharjee & Sharma, 2023). Family members often took for granted the presence of women at home, overlooking their work and increasing their responsibilities, with the expectation that they would always be available for domestic tasks, highlighting entrenched patriarchal attitudes (Bhat et al., 2022).

Banerjee and Wilks (2022) found that the pandemic heightened domestic control and surveillance, severely restricting women's mobility and autonomy. The sudden disruption of their ability to work or return home, exacerbated pre-existing patterns of patriarchal control as they had to renegotiate their autonomy and limited mobility, leading to feelings of claustrophobia, loss of control, and increased emotional stress.

As the men in the family exerted subtle to overt dominance over the women's lives and the lockdown guaranteed higher privacy and little to no way for the women to escape, there has also been a disturbing rise in instances of domestic violence and sexual abuse (Maji et al., 2022; Sumalatha et al., 2021). Literature suggests that this may be due to men displacing their frustrations over joblessness, wage reductions, alcohol non-availability, and other pandemic-related stresses onto vulnerable women in their homes (Tripathi et al., 2022). Bhat et al. (2022) observed that many WDWs, conditioned by patriarchal norms, felt it was their duty to endure such abuse, underlining the urgent need for sensitisation, support, and intervention. The authors also highlight the deep-seated gender inequalities within families, noting how financial strains often led families to sacrifice women's assets, like selling their jewellery, rather than male-held assets, exacerbating the women's long-term vulnerability and financial insecurity.

Thus, the intersection of amplified domestic responsibilities, patriarchal control, and the lack of social and legal support systems has created a challenging environment that requires targeted interventions to alleviate the burdens faced by these women.

Navigating the Post-Pandemic Terrain: Challenges So Far

In the aftermath of the COVID-19 pandemic, WDWs in India find themselves at a critical juncture, facing a myriad of challenges due to both systemic and interpersonal limitations, yet forging ahead with resilience. Drawing on the findings from the studies discussed thus far, this section delves into the multifaceted dimensions of their post-pandemic reality, underscoring the need for a comprehensive approach to address their concerns and bolster their wellbeing.

WDWs constitute a vital segment of India's socio-economic fabric, yet they are 'unrewarded by the society and unprotected by the state' (Banerjee & Wilks, 2022, p. 7). Despite their significant contribution to the economy, they continue to grapple with part-time employment, extended work hours, significant hurdles to upward mobility, and a lack of formal and legal protection and employment rights (Sharma, 2022). The pandemic has exacerbated these issues, with many workers facing job insecurity, reduced wages, and the absence of social security, amplifying their socio-economic vulnerabilities (Raval & Nizami, 2024). The situation is further compounded by the intersection of gender inequality, and caste and class-based stigma and discrimination limiting their bargaining power and subjecting them to the threat of job loss and non-payment of wages. However, the state of their vulnerability was largely ignored in the government's pandemic responses as the focus was largely on a biomedical perspective that prioritised curtailing the spread of the virus through 'social distancing', but failed to consider the socio-economic implications these public health measures would have on the most marginalised and poor (Thomas et al., 2021). Thus, for informal sector workers including WDWs, the public health guidelines served as forms of exclusion.

Further, the few measures taken by the government, like the appeal for employers to pay full wages to permanent and contractual workers during the pandemic lacked legal enforcement, leaving many workers at the mercy of individual employers (Singh & Kaur, 2022). Some scholars argue that the relief measures introduced by the government have been highly inadequate (Ghosh, 2020).

Additionally, a large body of research has established that the pandemic has disproportionately affected women more than men (Afridi et al., 2021; Jasrotia & Meena, 2021). However, the gendered impact has not been adequately addressed by existing policies and public health measures. The lack of gender-segregated data and gender analysis in pandemic interventions has not only obscured the gendered realities from empirical data but also hindered the development of inclusive post-pandemic policies (Agarwal, 2021). Mahanta & Gupta (2019) pointed out that such disaggregated data do not feature in most of the statistical standards and definitions of domestic work in India. This reflects the current lack of understanding and recognition, even at a policy level, of the structural discrimination they face, thus excluding them from getting legislative and policy-level protection.

It also must be noted that the experiences of WDWs vary across different regions and states in India, likely stemming from several socio-political variations. Along with city-wise differences in government response and aid to informal workers (Mohan et al., 2022), the existing social and economic network of the women also mattered. For instance, in Kerala, WDWs significantly benefitted from pre-existing government initiatives like Kudumbashree, a social and economic initiative to empower women implemented by the Kerala government, which strengthened their social networks and community engagement (George & Nandhini, 2024; Varghese & Rajan, 2012). However, research from other parts of India like Uttar Pradesh (see Sahoo, 2023) also points out that while workers accessed basic government facilities, they often remained unaware of or unable to access specific welfare schemes designed for them. Across many states, particularly for migrants, WDWs frequently fall outside the scope of social security and relief measures, facing significant barriers to government assistance (Sumalatha et al., 2021).

Despite all the above factors, Mukherjee and Mukhopadhyay (2022) reported in their study on WDWs from Kolkata that a large proportion of their participants expressed contentment regarding their work and earnings, despite acknowledging their low social status. They suggest that this reflects a complex interplay of intrinsic rewards shaped by gendered social norms and the satisfaction derived from meeting their basic economic needs. Similarly, WDWs report that they value their employment as it helps them financially support their families, makes them independent and gains them respect as workers, despite the lack of job security and precarity associated with it (Kumar & Baliyan, 2023)

The Way Forward: Recognising the Value of Domestic Work and Empowering Workers

The path to recovery and empowerment for WDWs involves acknowledging domestic work as a vital economic activity and ensuring socio-economic security for all workers. Formulating policies that recognise the contributions of domestic workers to the Gross Domestic Product and providing them with formal rights and benefits are essential steps towards achieving gender equality and sustainable development goals (Anand, 2021).

Chen (2020) suggests that the COVID-19 pandemic presents an opportunity for social and policy-level changes that positively impact informal workers going forward. This necessitates a recognition of the value of informal work, their economic contribution, and ensuring the workers' rights to social and economic wellbeing. Chen (2020) also brings up the threat of negative reversal through the undoing of years of progress through pandemic-related disruptions. For instance, many state governments in India, like Madhya Pradesh and Uttar Pradesh, have introduced legal changes during the pandemic that compromise labour rights by extending work hours, weakening labour laws, and even banning trade unions (Bhuta, 2022; Sundar, 2020). Concurrently, there is empirical and literary evidence that increasing the formalisation of domestic workers through unions can enhance their bargaining power and facilitate the articulation of class and gender-based prejudices. For instance, Parpiani (2021) discusses the impact of the GhareluKamgaar Union, a neighbourhood-level Dalit domestic workers' union in Mumbai. Bringing informal sector workers under the umbrella of a workers' union has helped to reframe domestic work, serving as a platform to address their issues and engage in discussions focused on respect and dignity. Further, organisations like the Self-Employed Women's Association have been pivotal in educating workers about their rights and enhancing their social and occupational opportunities at grassroots levels, showing direct benefits for the workers (Ismail & Ogando, 2023).

Thomas et al. (2021) suggest that improving livelihood options through flexible loan systems and skills training is one way to empower otherwise vulnerable workers during and post the pandemic. This necessitates a level of formalisation of the occupation of domestic work, with survey data collected and policies and laws enacted to define and ensure their rights. However, efforts towards skill promotion alone without formulating and implementing adequate legislative measures also do not protect workers from exploitation (Sharma, 2022).

Thus, for India to realise the 2030 agenda and the Sustainable Development Goals, the government has to take notice and introduce measures to protect the poor and marginalised (Chen, 2020). Building on their resilience, closing systemic gaps, and implementing inclusive policies will be crucial in ensuring their well-being and recognition within the broader socio-economic framework.

Limitations and Future Directions

This narrative review is based on a relatively small number of studies, most of which are qualitative. This reflects the broader issue of limited research on WDWs in India, particularly in the context of the COVID-19 pandemic. Further, many of the included papers discussed similar and overlapping themes which made the process of extracting specific, distinct themes challenging. The lack of quantitative literature restricted any comparative or meta-analytic assessments and also the ability to identify broader patterns across different populations and settings. Only articles published in English were included, which may have omitted literature published in non-English language publications.

One limitation of the studies included in this review is the lack of a clear theoretical framework, which could have provided a stronger conceptual foundation for the research questions and data analysis. The absence of theoretical models might limit the depth of analysis and the ability to draw broader conclusions about the systemic issues affecting this population. Future research should include a broader range of methodologies, incorporate quantitative data, and engage with theoretical frameworks that focus on labour, gender, caste, and intersectionality, among others, which can add to the conceptual and theoretical backing of studies on this marginalised population.

Conclusion

The pandemic has brought to light the ongoing precarity and marginalisation of domestic workers, with the new challenges that research shows have unequivocally widened the gender, caste, and class gap and inequalities in India (Bhat et al., 2022). The outcomes for many women were dire, leading to a significant shift in their livelihoods. With the lockdown, the workers found themselves losing existing employment opportunities and their incomes, and with no choice but to seek alternative, often lower-paying jobs. This situation was often exacerbated by the loss of existing rented housing, leading to a hole in their savings and increased debts and loans, from which it would take years to recover. Migrant labourers faced the disintegration of the fragile roots they had established in urban centres. Moreover, these challenges were compounded by an increased stigma attached to their occupation, caste and class status, further marginalising these women and their families. The compounded stress from heightened domestic responsibilities, financial instability, and negotiating individual autonomy within patriarchal systems, has led to significant psychological distress, manifesting in behavioural responses such as increased stress, anxiety, restlessness, decreased sleep, and altered eating habits that persist even post-pandemic. WDWs continue to navigate limited access to healthcare and increased financial burdens associated with medical costs. There is a critical need for inclusive policies and support systems that address the unique challenges faced by these workers. In summary, navigating the post-pandemic landscape for WDWs in India requires the recognition of their value as workers and a multifaceted approach that addresses their economic, health, and social challenges.

Acknowledgement

The author expresses her deep gratitude to Amrita Deb for her guidance and support throughout this work, and to Sunanda P. K., who inspired this study

Conflict of Interest

The author has no competing interest to report.

Funding

This research did not receive any specific grant from funding agencies in the public, commercial, or not-for-profit sectors.

References

Abraham, R., Basole, A., & Kesar, S. (2022). Down and out? The gendered impact of the COVID-19 pandemic on India's labour market. *Economia Politica*, *39*(1), 101–128. https://doi.org/10.1007/s40888-021-00234-8

Afridi, F., Dhillon, A., & Roy, S. (2021). The *G*endered *C*risis: Livelihoods and *M*ental *W*ell-*B*eing in India during COVID-19 (Vol. 2021). UNU-WIDER. https://doi.org/10.35188/UNU-WIDER/2021/003-0

Agarwal, B. (2021). Reflections on the less visible and less measured: Gender and COVID-19 in India. *Gender & Society*, *35*(2), 244–255. https://doi.org/10.1177/08912432211001299

Alex, R., Sathish, K., & Jebaraj, P. (2022). Work related illness among female domestic workers employed in private homes in South India. *Safety and Health at Work*, *13*, S283. https://doi.org/10.1016/j.shaw.2021.12.1636

Allard, J., Jagnani, M., Neggers, Y., Pande, R., Schaner, S., & Moore, C. T. (2022). Indian female migrants face greater barriers to post-Covid recovery than males: Evidence from a panel study. *eClinicalMedicine*, *53*, 101631.https://doi.org/10.1016/j.eclinm.2022.101631

Anand, M. K. (2021). *COVID-19 and informal labour: A study of women domestic workers*. *9*(3). https://doi.org/10.25215/0903.178

Anusuya, G. S., Patki, M. B., Hruaii, V., Lalengkimi, R., Zuali, L., Marimuthu, K., Tochhawng, L., Zothanzama, J., Kumar, N. S., & Zuala, S. (2022). A study of rural domestic helpers knowledge, attitude, and practice of COVID-19 in Mizoram, India. *Asian Journal of Medical Sciences*, *13*(12), Article 12. https://doi.org/10.3126/ajms.v13i12.46069

Banerjee, S., & Wilks, L. (2022). Work in pandemic times: exploring precarious continuities in paid domestic work in India. *Gender, Work, and Organization*, 10.1111/gwao.12858. Advance online publication. https://doi.org/10.1111/gwao.12858

Bhargava, R., & Bhargava, M. (2021, June 15). COVID-19 *I*s *C*reating a *H*unger *C*atastrophe in India – *H*ere's an *O*pportunity to *B*reak the *C*ycle. World Economic Forum. www.weforum.org/agenda/2021/06/covid-19-pandemic-hunger-catastrophe-india-poverty-food-insecurity-relief/

Bhat, L., Kandaswamy, S., Sumalatha, B. S., Mohan, G., & Tatsi, O. (2022). Fear, discrimination, and healthcare access during the COVID-19 pandemic: Exploring women domestic workers' lives in India. *Agenda*, *35*, 1–11. https://doi.org/10.1080/10130950.2021.2046392

Bhattacharjee, S., & Goswami, B. (2020). Female domestic workers: income determinants and empowerment correlates–a case study. *The Indian Journal of Labour Economics*, *63*(2), 483–498. https://doi.org/10.1007/s41027-020-00223-8

Bhattacharjee, S., & Sharma, M. (2023). A gendered approach to examining pandemic-induced livelihood crisis in the informal sector: the case of female domestic workers in Titwala. In *The Role of GIS in COVID-19 Management and Control*(1st ed., p. 263). CRC Press. https://doi.org/10.1201/9781003227106

Bhattacharya, D., Sukumar, M., & Mani, M. (2016). *Living on the Margins: A Study of Domestic Workers in Chennai, India*. Centre for Workers' Management. Accessed at www.academia.edu/65484268/Living_on_the_Margins_A_Study_of_Domestic_Workers_in_Chennai

Bhuta, A. (2022). Imbalancing act: India's Industrial Relations Code, 2020. *The Indian Journal of Labour Economics*, *65*(3), 821–830. https://doi.org/10.1007/s41027-022-00389-3

Chadha, N. (2020). *Domestic Workers in India: An Invisible Workforce. Issue Brief.* Social Policy Research Foundation.

Chen, M. (2020). COVID-19, Cities and urban informal workers: India in comparative perspective. *The Indian Journal of Labour Economics*, *63*(S1), 41–46. https://doi.org/10.1007/s41027-020-00254-1

Choolayil, A. C., & Putran, L. (2021). The COVID-19 pandemic and human dignity: The case of migrant labourers in India. *Journal of Human Rights and Social Work*, *6*(3), 225–236. https://doi.org/10.1007/s41134-021-00185-x

Daraei, M., & Mohajery, A. (2013). The impact of socio-economic status on life satisfaction. *Social Indicators Research*, *112*(1), 69–81. https://doi.org/10.1007/s11205-012-0040-x

Dasgupta, J., & Mitra, S. (2020, May 30). A gender-responsive policy and fiscal response to the pandemic. *Economic and Political Weekly*, *55*(22), 7–8.

Deshpande, A. (2020). The Covid-19 pandemic and lockdown: First order effects on gender gaps in employment and domestic time use in India. GLO Discussion Paper, *No. 607. Global Labor Organization (GLO)*, Essen, www.econstor.eu/handle/10419/222416

Dey, A. K., Bhan, N., Rao, N., Ghule, M., Chatterji, S., & Raj, A. (2022). Factors affecting delayed and non-receipt of healthcare during the COVID-19 pandemic for women in rural Maharashtra, India: Evidence from a cross-sectional study. *eClinicalMedicine*, *53*, 1–12. https://doi.org/10.1016/j.eclinm.2022.101741

Dickey, S. (2000). Permeable homes: Domestic service, household space, and the vulnerability of class boundaries in urban India. *American Ethnologist*, *27*(2), 462–489. https://doi.org/10.1525/ae.2000.27.2.462

Estupinan, X., & Sharma, M. (2020). Job and wage losses in informal sector due to the COVID-19 lockdown measures in India. *SSRN Electronic Journal*. https://doi.org/10.2139/ssrn.3680379

George, A., & Nandhini, D. M. (2024). A study on work-life quality of female domestic workers. *International Journal for Multidisciplinary Research*, *6*(1), 1–9. https://doi.org/10.36948/ijfmr.2024.v06i01.10380

Ghatak, A., & Sarkar, K. (2022). The impact of the COVID-19 pandemic on domestic workers in India. In *COVID-19 Pandemic, Public Policy, and Institutions in India*. Routledge. https://doi.org/10.4324/9781003226970

Ghosh, J. (2020). A critique of the Indian government's response to the COVID-19 pandemic. *Journal of Industrial and Business Economics*, *47*(3), 519–530. https://doi.org/10.1007/s40812-020-00170-x

Gupta, S., Das, D., Bhattacharya, S. K., & Gupta, S. S. (2022). How COVID-19 affected the work prospects and healthcare-seeking of women domestic workers in Kolkata City, India? A longitudinal study. *Indian Journal of Occupational and Environmental Medicine*, *26*(3), 157. https://doi.org/10.4103/ijoem.ijoem_346_21

International Labour Organization. (2010). About *D*omestic *W*ork. www.ilo.org/resource/about-domestic-work

International Labour Organization. (2018, April 30). Women and *M*en in the *I*nformal *E*conomy: A *S*tatistical *P*icture (3rd ed.). www.ilo.org/publications/women-and-men-informal-economy-statistical-picture-third-edition

Ismail, G., & Ogando, A. C. (2023, February). *Domestic Workers during the COVID-19 Crisis: Pathways of Impact, Recovery, and Resilience in Six Cities. WIEGO Resource Document No. 31.* www.wiego.org/sites/default/files/publications/file/wiego-resource-document-No.31.pdf

Jasrotia, A., & Meena, J. (2021). Women, work and pandemic: An impact study of COVID-19 lockdown on working women in India. *Asian Social Work and Policy Review*, *15*(3), 282–291. https://doi.org/10.1111/aswp.12240

Jesline, J., Romate, J., Rajkumar, E., & George, A. J. (2021). The plight of migrants during COVID-19 and the impact of circular migration in India: A systematic review. *Humanities and Social Sciences Communications*, *8*(1), 1–12. https://doi.org/10.1057/s41599-021-00915-6

Jha, S. S., & Lahiri, A. (2020). Domestic migrant workers in India returning to their homes: Emerging socio-economic and health challenges during the COVID-19 pandemic. *Rural and Remote Health*, *20*(4), 6186. https://doi.org/10.22605/RRH6186

Khillare, P. Y., & Sonawane, M. A. (2016). The impact of work-life of women domestic workers on their family-life. *IOSR Journal of Business and Management*, *18*(08), 47–50. https://doi.org/10.9790/487X-1808024750

Kujur, S. K., & Goswami, D. (2020). COVID-19: Severity of the pandemic and responses of Indian states. *Journal of Public Affairs*, *20*(4), e2362. https://doi.org/10.1002/pa.2362

Kumar, N. P., & Baliyan, K. (2023). The impact of the COVID-19 pandemic on female domestic workers in an urban setting. In Fazli, A. & Kundu, A. (Eds.), *Reimagining Prosperity: Social and Economic Development in Post-COVID India* (pp. 259–281). Palgrave Macmillan Singapore. https://doi.org/10.1007/978-981-19-7177-8_15

Mahanta, U., & Gupta, I. (2019). Introducing the status of domestic workers in India. In U. Mahanta & I. Gupta (Eds.), *Recognition of the Rights of Domestic Workers in India* (pp. 1–17). Springer Singapore. https://doi.org/10.1007/978-981-13-5764-0_1

Maji, S., Bansod, S., & Singh, T. (2022). Domestic violence during COVID-19 pandemic: The case for Indian women. *Journal of Community & Applied Social Psychology*, *32*(3), 374–381. https://doi.org/10.1002/casp.2501

Ministry of Labour & Employment. (2023, August 3). *Condition of Domestic Workers*. https://pib.gov.in/pib.gov.in/Pressreleaseshare.aspx?PRID=1945512

Mohan, D., Sekhani, R., Mistry, J., Mishra, S., Singh, A., Mittal, V., Pachauri, R., Chindaliyan, S., & Mohan, T. (2022). Gauging the impact of a pandemic on the lives and livelihoods of female domestic worker across Indian cities. *International Journal of Health Sciences*, 11653–11672. https://doi.org/10.53730/ijhs.v6nS3.8784

Mukherjee, T., & Mukhopadhyay, I. (2022). Albeit satisfied: Unveiling female paid domestic workers in India. *Indian Journal of Human Development*, *16*(2), 248–266. https://doi.org/10.1177/09737030221123189

National Domestic Workers' Movement. (n.d.). Domestic Workers – NDWM – The National Domestic Workers' Movement. Retrieved May 30, 2024, from https://ndwm.org/domestic-workers/

Neetha, N. (2009). Contours of domestic service: Characteristics, work relations and regulations. *The Indian Journal of Labour Economics*, *52*(3), 489–506. https://idwfed.org/en/resources/contours-of-domestic-service-characteristics-work-relations-and-regulations

Parpiani, M. (2021). Becoming working class: Domestic workers and the claim to localness in Mumbai. *Anthropology of Work Review*, *42*(2), 120–130. https://doi.org/10.1111/awr.12225

Pinchoff, J., Santhya, K. G., White, C., Rampal, S., Acharya, R., & Ngo, T. D. (2020). Gender specific differences in COVID-19 knowledge, behavior and health effects among adolescents and young adults in Uttar Pradesh and Bihar, India. *PLOS ONE*, *15*(12), e0244053. https://doi.org/10.1371/journal.pone.0244053

Ramani, S., Bahuguna, M., Tiwari, A., Shende, S., Waingankar, A., Sridhar, R., Shaikh, N., Das, S., Pantvaidya, S., Fernandez, A., & Jayaraman, A. (2022). Corona was scary, lockdown was worse: A mixed-methods study of community perceptions on COVID-19 from urban informal settlements of Mumbai. *PLOS ONE, 17*(5), e0268133. https://doi.org/10.1371/journal.pone.0268133

Raval, G., & Nizami, N. (2024). Current status of decent work for female domestic workers in India. *SSRN Electronic Journal*. https://doi.org/10.2139/ssrn.4696098

Raveendran, G., & Vanek, J. (2020, August). *Current Status of Decent Work for Female Domestic Workers in India*. Women in Informal Employment: Globalizing and Organizing. www.wiego.org/publications/informal-workers-india-statistical-profile

Sahni, S. P., & Junnarkar, M. (2019). 'Well-being' of domestic workers in India. In U. Mahanta & I. Gupta (Eds.), *Recognition of the Rights of Domestic Workers in India: Challenges and the Way Forward* (pp. 163–175). Springer. https://doi.org/10.1007/978-981-13-5764-0_9

Sahoo, A. (2023). Profiles in female poverty: The invisible domestic workers. *International Journal for Multidisciplinary Research, 5*(3), 6290. https://doi.org/10.36948/ijfmr.2023.v05i03.6290

Seedat-Khan, M., Dharmaraja, G., & Sidloyi, S. (2014). A new form of bonded labour: A comparative study between domestic workers of South Africa and India. *Journal of Sociology and Social Anthropology, 4*, 31–40. www.researchgate.net/profile/Mariam-Seedat-Khan/publication/273682487_A_New_Form_of_Bonded_Labour_A_Comparative_Study_between_Domestic_Workers_of_South_Africa_and_India/links/5e43be97a6fdccd9659be218/A-New-Form-of-Bonded-Labour-A-Comparative-Study-between-Domestic-Workers-of-South-Africa-and-India.pdf

Sharma, S. (2022). Domestic workers, class-hegemony, and the Indian state: A sociological perspective on ideology. *South Asian History and Culture, 13*(4), 528–545. https://doi.org/10.1080/19472498.2022.2068481

Singh, N., & Kaur, A. (2022). The COVID-19 pandemic: Narratives of informal women workers in Indian Punjab. *Gender, Work & Organization, 29*(2), 388–407. https://doi.org/10.1111/gwao.12766

Sumalatha, B. S., Bhat, L. D., & Chitra, K. P. (2021). Impact of Covid-19 on informal sector: A study of women domestic workers in India. *The Indian Economic Journal, 69*(3), 441–461. https://doi.org/10.1177/00194662211023845

Sundar, K. R. S. (2020). COVID-19 and state failure: A double whammy for trade unions and labour rights. *The Indian Journal of Labour Economics, 63*(Suppl 1), 97–103. https://doi.org/10.1007/s41027-020-00263-0

Thomas, J., de, W. E. E., Radhakrishnan, R. K., Kulkarni, N., & Bunders-Aelen, J. G. F. (2021). Mitigating the COVID-19 pandemic in India: An in-depth exploration of challenges and opportunities for three vulnerable population groups. *Equality, Diversity and Inclusion: An International Journal, 41*(1), 49–63. https://doi.org/10.1108/EDI-09-2020-0264

Tripathi, P., Dwivedi, P., & Sharma, S. (2022). Psychological impact of domestic violence on women in India due to COVID-19. *International Journal of Human Rights in Healthcare, 16*(2), 146–161. https://doi.org/10.1108/IJHRH-12-2021-0208

Ugargol, A. P., & Parvathy, L. (2022). Precarity of informal work, absence of social security, and ageism: The persistence of social inequalities and challenges for older adults' labor force participation in India. In Rajan, S. I. (Ed.), *Handbook of Aging, Health and Public Policy: Perspectives from Asia* (pp. 1–29). Springer Singapore. https://doi.org/10.1007/978-981-16-1914-4_173-1

Varghese, V. J., & Rajan, S. I. (2012). Governmentality, social stigma, and quasi-citizenship: Gender negotiations of migrant women domestic workers from Kerala. In Rajan, S. I., & Percot, M. (Eds.), *Dynamics of Indian Migration: Historical and Current Perspectives* (pp. 224–248). Routledge India. https://doi.org/10.4324/9780367818043

Waghmore, S., & Contractor, Q. (2015). On the madness of caste: Dalits; Muslims; and normalized incivilities in neoliberal India. In Mohan, B. (Ed.), *Global Frontiers of Social Development in Theory and Practice* (pp. 223–240). Palgrave Macmillan New York. https://doi.org/10.1057/9781137460714_12

World Health Organisation (WHO). (2020). Impact of COVID-19 on People's Livelihoods, their Health and our Food Systems. www.who.int/news/item/13-10-2020-impact-of-covid-19-on-people's-livelihoods-their-health-and-our-food-systems

8 Neuro-Divergence and COVID-19 Pandemic

A Reflexive Thematic Analysis on the Experiences of a Mother of an Autistic Child

Sonali Mukherjee and Swati Pathak

Introduction

The neurodiversity movement has gained momentum in recent decades, emphasising autism as a human rights issue rather than a collection of deficits and challenges (Kapp, 2020). This perspective advocates for the inclusion and autonomy of neuro-divergent individuals and promotes parental acceptance of autism through exposure to neurodiversity viewpoints (Cascio, 2015).

A progressive shift in understanding and conceptualising autism has taken place from viewing autism embedded in the conventional medical paradigm to focusing on the interplay between contextual and individual factors and comprehending the priorities of the neuro-divergent community (Pelicano & Houting, 2022). People across the autism spectrum and their parents who serve as non-autistic allies are seen as diverse individuals who are a part of the neurodiversity movement, to provide a full range of developmental experiences with acceptance, support, and dignity in society, rather than dehumanising and reducing the identities of people with autism. The inclusion of caregivers and allies in the development of autism research is essential, to engage and steer interventions and to humanise this process by moving beyond historical misrepresentation of people with neuro-divergence (Leadbitter et al., 2021). The COVID-19 pandemic brought to reality the masked inequalities present in the space of the mental health spectrum and revealed significant difficulties and challenges presented to neuro-divergent individuals including exclusion from accessing resources of care, prolonged isolation, lack of support networks as well as economic inequalities (Pellicano et al., 2020). Navigating parenthood under these circumstances posed immense challenges, especially for those with children requiring special attention. The closure of special education services resulted in a profound loss of essential support systems, leaving parents to shoulder the responsibilities of full-time caregiving alone. Many found themselves thrust into a daunting role for which they often lacked the necessary skills and resources to navigate effectively (Tokatly, 2021). These issues further highlighted the urgent need to make the health system more sensitive towards children's health and thereby cater to neuro-divergent children (Jansen et al., 2022).

DOI: 10.4324/9781003517313-9

History of Autism and Neurodiversity

Brief Overview of Developments in Autism

Since the inception and development of psychology, the question of what is normal and what is not has been central to understanding and furthering knowledge of human behaviour. Advancements in the field further brought disagreements among members of the field, considering the socio-cultural, intersectional, and political issues at hand, which served as groundbreaking factors due to which the binary of normal–abnormal started being questioned. Kanner (1943) described autism as a result of emotionally cold parenting, known as refrigerator parenting (Cohmer, 2014). In contrast, Hans Asperger took a strengths-based approach, focusing on creating supportive environments for differently wired individuals, a concept highlighted by Lorna Wing, who named it Asperger's syndrome to broaden understanding of the autism spectrum (Lai & Baron-Cohen, 2015; Watts, 2014). However, Sheffer (2018) raised controversies about Asperger's work, pointing out its eugenic and Nazi connotations. From Kanner (1943) describing autism as a product of emotional cold and lack of parental warmth, due to the result of refrigerator parenting (Cohmer, 2014), to Hans Asperger following a strengths-based approach in creating an environment well-suited for differently wired individuals, this, following a strengths-based approach rather than solely focusing on their difficulties (Lai & Baron-Cohen, 2015) whose seminal work was first brought to light by Lorna Wing who felt motivated to broaden the understanding of the autism spectrum by using the founder's eponym and thereby naming it as Asperger's syndrome (Watts, 2014) with further controversies raised on the intent and goodwill of Hans Asperger's work as laid down by Sheffer (2018) who pointed out the eugenist and Nazi connotations in Asperger's work while catering to autistic children in his clinic. Refrigerator mother was a controversial theory proposed in the mid-20th century, suggesting that autism in children was caused by emotionally cold and distant mothers. This theory, popularised by psychiatrist Leo Kanner (1943), placed blame on mothers for their children's autistic behaviours, asserting that a lack of maternal warmth and affection led to the development of autism (Cohmer, 2014).

Rise of Neurodiversity Movement

The term neurodiversity was conceptualised by Judy Singer in 1998, a sociologist with autism spectrum disorder, to bring a dynamic shift from the deficit-oriented discourse on cognitive variations towards diversity-oriented perspectives on understanding atypical ways of thinking (Silberman, 2017). Singer's purpose was to create a foundation for the autistic culture to come together, to build a steady ground for the autistic self-advocacy movement (Doyle et al., 2022), and to understand the true nature of neurodiversity (Singer, 1998). A book titled *Nothing About Us, Without Us: Disability, Oppression and Empowerment* written by James I. Charlton (1998) elucidates the resistance towards disability oppression as part of the disability rights movement as a way of self-determination for the disabled population. This book is considered as a classic text in the landscape of disability rights advocacy. However, as the growth of the neurodiversity movement took place, more autistic self-advocates started realising the exclusion of neuro-diverse narratives from the larger disability discussion (Hughes, 2016). A revolutionary and influential essay titled 'Don't Mourn For Us' by Jim Sinclair in 1999 is an undoubtedly important piece in the autistic people's advocacy movement and in shaping the history of neurodiversity. Sinclair noted the parental tendency to direct grief towards their child's autistic identity and also acknowledged that their grief is real and natural due to the cultural assumptions for parents to have a 'normal child' but also urged parents to not mourn for their child, as he noted, 'You didn't lose a child to autism. You lost a child because the child you waited for never came into existence' (Pripas, 2020, p. 34). 'Grieve if you must, for your lost dreams. But don't mourn for us. We are alive. We are real. And we're here waiting for you' (Sinclair, 1999, p. 3). Sinclair's essay paved the way forward from shifting the perception of autism as a tragedy towards empowering the autistic self-advocacy movement to reshape expectations and norms around autism imposed by society (Kapit, 2020).

Social Model of Disability

Previously, there were several competing models of disability that not only provided different notions of disability but also determined how disabilities impact individuals' wellbeing (Jurgens, 2021). Among all the models of disability, the most orthodox model is the medical model, it views physical or cognitive differences primarily as disabilities, which are classified as functional deficits or dysfunctions that an individual either has or does not have (Olkin, 2002). This model conceptualises differences as deficits that need correction, leading to intervention strategies focused mainly on disabled individuals. In this sense, disability is directly associated with deficit or dysfunction, diverging from what is considered normal functioning. Critics, such as Blume (1998), Singer (1999), Chown and Beavan (2012), Armstrong (2015), and Chapman (2019a), have labelled this as a default pathologisation of disability and neurodivergence. They argue that this approach inherently frames disability and neurodivergence as deviations from an established norm, thus emphasising the need for correction rather than acceptance or accommodation. The lens through which autism is viewed has changed over the past decades. The shift from the neurodiversity paradigm is embedded in the framework of the social model of disability which implies that the disability does not lie within the individual but rather in the social norms, barriers, and structures within the society with a distinction between individual limitations and social disablement (Chapman, 2019). However, this model has met with much criticism and scrutiny within autism research over the years. Mike Oliver (1983), one of the originators of the social model of disability, intended to empower disabled people by focusing light on the social obstacles faced by the community as an academic–political instrument and not to replace the medical model of disability (Kapp, 2019). Further discourse on reinvigorating the social model of autism by Levitt (2017) while commenting on the work, Oliver (2013) identified the need for the social model to be reflective of the social conditions in the geographical regions in which it is used, while Woods (2017) further commented on the need for the social model to be implemented through bringing change through shifting non-autistic people's attitudes towards autism through inclusion of positive language for autism along with the enactment of laws for autism.

Definitions of Neurodiversity and Linguistic Preferences of the Neuro-Diverse Community

The language of neurodiversity has been developed from the inputs of several contributors who have made efforts to bring to light important terms and terminologies to understand diversity in an informed manner.

It must also be noted that the historical misrepresentation of the autistic community has been prevalent in the use of language to describe autistic people. Language plays an important role in either the reduction or perpetuation of stigma (Bottema-Buetel et al., 2021) within disability narratives. This can be highlighted in the debate between Identity-First Language (IFL) and Person-First Language (PFL) with no clear consensus about the most favourable or preferred language to represent the autistic community (Vivanti, 2020). It is reflected in the current literature that the usage of both IFL and PFL are acceptable in varied contexts by different groups and communities (Taboas et al., 2023; Buijsman et al., 2023; Bury et al., 2023; Kenny et al., 2016).

Narratives of Caregivers with Neuro-Divergent Children

Parental voices have been instrumental in questioning and illuminating nuanced perspectives and inclusive discourses on autism (Langan, 2011). Observing the importance of the process of advocacy for children with autism, parents have served as one of the most central tenets in revolutionising the perception and attitude towards autistic children by the criticism brought upon to the now obsolete concept of refrigerator mothers and to become empowered advocates for their children (Cleary et al., 2023).

The invisibility and underrepresentation of the narratives of the caregivers of children with autism are quite prevalent in the existing literature in India. The engagement of parents is of significant importance in catering to the needs of neuro-divergent children. Their involvement is important in identifying the cognitive, physiological, and behavioural patterns of the child, which require support and intervention (Agazzi et al., 2019). Parents also serve as a bridge between the home and other schooling environments of the child (Prata et al., 2018) and in the process, also become co-therapists in collaboration with therapists in factors such as early diagnosis and therapy, the psychological wellbeing of caregivers, participating in training, group support, and management programs to enable the parents to develop and learn behavioural management skills, to mitigate the burden of intensive therapy from a parent-mediated framework (Kotsopoulou et al., 2021; Rajaraman & Mundkur, 2021; Hassenfeldt, 2015).

The stigmas associated with autism are not only found in diagnostic labels and their underlying prejudices but also towards the perception of the mother–child unit in societies, wherein mothers are not seen as independently functioning individuals (Swanke et al, 2009).

Preliminary Information

Background: The present study delves into the experiences of a mother, aged 43, whose son was diagnosed with autism spectrum disorder (ASD) at the age of 4 in 2011. The mother, who got married at the age of 25 and became a parent at the age of 27 in 2008, encountered immense challenges upon receiving the diagnosis, particularly grappling with its impact. Despite initial devastation, the parents embarked on a journey of acceptance and actively sought therapies for their child, including speech and occupational therapy, as well as specialised education. The socioeconomic status of the family is upper middle class (as per the scores obtained on the parameters of education and occupation described in the modified Kuppuswamy socioeconomic scale, 2023) where both parents were working. However, after the child was diagnosed with autism, the mother left the job, since there was little support system from the family.

Family, medical and developmental history: As per the interviewer (mother), the couple had an arranged marriage and did not have any health issues. The family is a nuclear family, living in their own house. The child under study is the only child of the couple. Mother's health during pregnancy was good and she did not face any major psychological stressors during the entire pregnancy period. The father is healthy and is not diagnosed with any physical or mental illness. The paternal grandmother has diabetes. Mother was diagnosed with sclerosis in the year 2012. Apart from these, there is no known history of any other illness in the family.

Proceeding with a description of prenatal and birth history, the mother had a normal pregnancy and attended all antenatal clinics regularly. The child was born by lower segment caesarean section after a complete 9 months of gestation when the mother did not have natural labour around the expected date of delivery. At birth, the child did not cry immediately, was pale, and had to be shifted to the Intensive Care Unit (ICU). The child's Apgar score is unknown and his birth weight was 2.5 kg. The child remained in the ICU for a few days and during those days, mother had to provide the breast milk via breast pump to the nurse which was later fed to the child.

The mother further stated that the child's motor milestones were attained within the normal period. The social milestones including speech were delayed. The child did not maintain eye contact with the mother or any other individual. The child was examined by the family physician and was reported to have a delay in growth and development.

The psychological assessments of the child were conducted by a clinical psychologist at Government hospital in paediatric department located in Delhi which included the Vineland Social Maturity Scale (VSMS), Gessel Drawing Test (GDT), NIMHANS SLD Battery, and Childhood Autism Rating Scale. On VSMS, the child has a social age of 7 years 7 months and an intelligence quotient of 84, indicative of 'dull average' functioning in the social area. The other evaluations showed that the child's overall cognitive abilities fell into the 'dull average' range with an IQ of 88 on GDT. Further, the child also displayed signs of mild to moderate ASD.

According to the mother, the child, at present, uses technology (cell phone and television) as per his interest without much assistance. The child enjoys listening to music. He is taken out with family members for family occasions and recreational outings and has been known to adapt with considerable ease.

Management: The child underwent various therapies like occupational therapy and speech therapy. Special educational inputs, specially targeted at improving the child's comprehension and thinking skills were taken. Occupational therapy and sensory integration therapy, as recommended by the clinical psychologist, were instrumental in overcoming sensory issues and stimulating the developmental process. The child's reaction to these therapies was positive, showing gradual improvement in handling sensory input and participating more comfortably in everyday activities. Speech therapy was also an integral part of the child's intervention plan, focusing on enhancing communication skills. The child initially showed some resistance to these sessions, often feeling frustrated, but with consistent support, they began to engage more willingly, resulting in noticeable progress in expressive and receptive language abilities. To further support the child's social development, group-based interactions were incorporated into the therapy regimen. At first, the child was hesitant and found it difficult to interact with peers, but over time, these sessions helped them become more socially engaged and better at forming connections with others. The child was admitted to an integrated school after diagnosis and followed a structural program that was carried out both at school and at home. In the school, he is eligible for scribe and compensatory time as per the Central Board of Secondary Education rule for students with learning disability. As the family has seen improvement in his condition with occupational therapy and speech therapy, the mother also enrolled herself in a 1-year certificate course on autism, to better understand and manage the child's condition and also to deepen her understanding and better support her child. This proactive step was driven by the visible improvements seen in the child's condition following the consistent application of occupational and speech therapies.

COVID-19 Pandemic Time

The mother described the pandemic period to be a difficult time for the family and the child as the entire routine was disrupted. Changes in routine lead to changes in behaviour and hence working on a new routine and bringing it into action was required for the benefit of the child.

Objective

The objective of the present study was to explore the experiences concerning challenges and opportunities of the mother of an autistic child during the COVID-19 pandemic outbreak.

Rationale

The author's decision to focus on this single case is driven by the profound commitment and dedication exhibited by the mother, making it a compelling subject for in-depth analysis. This case exemplifies the extraordinary measures taken by a parent in the face of multifaceted challenges. Various previous researches have pointed out that parents of children with ASD experience a higher level of parenting stress as compared to parents of children without any developmental disabilities (DDs) and parents of children with other types of DDs (Estes et al., 2009; Hayes & Watson, 2013; Rodriguez et al., 2019). The mother's perseverance in managing her own health condition, sclerosis, while simultaneously navigating the complexities of raising a child with autism, highlights the intersection of personal and caregiving stressors. In the studies conducted by Soltanifar et al., (2015), it was found that mothers experience greater levels of parental stress than fathers. Similarly in a retrospective study in Saudi Arabia, the researchers concluded that the level of depression was significantly higher among mothers of children with ASD than among mothers of children with typical development. In the same line, a study conducted in Iran using a small sample size found high levels of anxiety among mothers of children with ASD (Vilaseca, Ferrer, & Olmos, 2014).

In the present study, mother's proactive approach during the COVID-19 pandemic—where many support systems were disrupted—further underscores her exceptional resilience and resourcefulness. She adapted to the new circumstances by learning and implementing new strategies to support her child's educational and developmental needs, ensuring continuity in his progress despite external adversities.

Method

A single case study approach was employed for the present study (*N* = 1), wherein a qualitative approach was adopted, featuring an in-depth interview with the mother residing in New Delhi. Conducted in July 2023, the interview consisted of 10 open-ended questions (Appendix) derived from a semi-structured guide tailored for this study. The transcription of the interview was done using Otter software. In addition, Smail's (2005) power mapping technique was used to help structure the interview schedule in terms of the areas that were intended to be explored when interviewing the participant (e.g., family relationships, educational and developmental support, healthcare and therapeutic support, personal experience, and wellbeing).

This case not only sheds light on the specific challenges faced by parents of children with autism but also illustrates broader themes of resilience, adaptability, and the impact of parental involvement on child development. The depth of the mother's commitment offers valuable insights into the personal sacrifices and innovative solutions employed by caregivers in similar situations. Thus, this single case study serves as a powerful narrative that can inform and inspire both researchers and practitioners in the fields of psychology, education, and special needs care.

Informed consent, was obtained via telephone recording before the interview, and also debriefing was done. The interview was conducted in English with one of the authors being the interviewer. To mitigate any biases, both authors engaged in regular reflexive journaling and discussions with experts to critically examine their perspectives and assumptions. This included reflecting on how their research experiences shaped their understanding of the participants' experiences and being open to alternative interpretations. By incorporating these reflexive practices, the researchers aim to produce a nuanced and balanced understanding of the experiences of mothers of autistic children, acknowledging the complex interplay of family dynamics, educational and medical support, social and community involvement, economic factors, and personal wellbeing.

For analysis, Reflexive Thematic Analysis was employed to extract the essence of the participant's responses, categorising them into key themes. The inductive approach was utilised to analyse the narrative obtained as it allows the data to speak for itself, without the influence of any preconceived notions. With this approach, the researcher looks at the data and derives patterns and themes that can be used to explain the story. The analysis is based on Braun and Clarke's (2006) framework that includes six steps: (1) familiarising with data, (2) creating codes, (3) creating themes, (4) reviewing themes, (5) defining themes, and (6) writing a research report.

Positionality and Reflexivity Information on the Authors

The first author's area of research is neurodevelopmental disorder where she majorly dealt with children diagnosed with dyslexia. With a background of experience in neurodevelopmental disorders, she has extensive experience working with children with autism and their families in various therapeutic and educational settings. She also served as a school counsellor for 4.5 years catering majorly to children's emotional and developmental needs. The second author has a doctorate in psychology, having experience working with cervix cancer clients during her doctoral work. Her research interest also lies in family and couples therapy and gender and sexuality. She has served as a counsellor at a private setup and has dealt with the emotional issues of children and their parents.

Results

The reflexive thematic analysis of the interview with the mother of an autistic child during the COVID-19 pandemic revealed a rich tapestry of experiences, emotions, and challenges. Through her narrative, six salient themes emerged, offering profound insights into the complexities of parenting a child with autism amidst unprecedented circumstances.

Theme 1: Resilience in Adversity

The mother's narrative illuminated her resilience in the face of adversity. Despite the initial shock and devastation upon receiving her child's diagnosis, she displayed remarkable strength in embracing the challenges head-on. Throughout the pandemic, she exhibited unwavering determination to ensure her child's wellbeing, seeking out resources, therapies, and support networks through virtual platforms (scheduling meetings with therapists; and other parents whose children had similar diagnoses) to navigate the uncharted waters of autism.

> Despite the challenges, I am committed to providing the best possible support for my child with autism. Each day presents new hurdles, but my determination to adapt and learn alongside my child fuels my resilience. It's a journey of constant growth and discovery. The pandemic was the time when I became more determined to provide support to my child. Though it was very difficult initially as there was an entire change in not only my child's routine but my entire family's routine became upside down. That's when I realised that I couldn't completely depend on external support. I should myself also learn a few skills to help my child's growth. I felt I couldn't just let go of all of the hard work done till date for my child.

Theme 2: Struggles with Social Isolation and Educational Support

The participant vividly expressed the heightened sense of social isolation experienced by herself, her child, and the family as a whole during the pandemic. With disruptions to routine therapies, school closures, and limited social interactions, her child grappled with increased frustration and a sense of disconnect from the world around him. The mother experienced feelings of being stuck and vulnerable due to social isolation and a lack of support. Without an outlet to express her frustration and helplessness, she struggled with the insufficient skills needed to support her child during the pandemic. The mother's narrative underscored the profound impact of social isolation on her child's emotional and behavioural wellbeing, highlighting the urgent need for innovative solutions to mitigate its effects.

> During the pandemic, it felt like we were stranded on an island, isolated from the world. My son thrives on routine and structure, so when everything shut down, it was like his lifeline was suddenly cut off. His therapies were disrupted, school closed, and social interactions became almost nonexistent. He couldn't understand why everything had changed, and it broke my heart to see him struggle with frustration and confusion. It was like watching him drift further away from the world around him. We tried our best to create a sense of normalcy at home, but it was never the same. The isolation took a toll on his emotional and

> behavioural well-being, and it was a constant battle to keep his spirits up. We desperately need innovative solutions to help children like him navigate these challenging times and reconnect with the world.
>
> When there was a description in therapies and schools were closed, me and my family had to struggle to help my child with his studies. We were not so equipped with the skills to teach him or children like him, this thought of not being able to help my child used to make me feel helpless and guilty. It was impacting my wellbeing and peace of mind.

Theme 3: Adaptation and Creativity

Amidst the challenges posed by the pandemic, the mother demonstrated remarkable adaptability and creativity in meeting her child's evolving needs. From leveraging tele-therapy sessions to devising at-home learning activities tailored to her child's interests and abilities, she showcased a resourcefulness born out of love and dedication. Her narrative underscored the importance of flexibility and innovation in navigating the complexities of autism in a rapidly changing world.

> When faced with adversity, a new strength emerges from within. My entire family shares a special bond, an emotional connection that can overcome any challenge together. During the lockdown, I created a world of my own for my child. I filled his mind's eye with light, paving new paths through every difficulty. I remember my mother in law telling me one day that there is no greater power than a mother's love, no test too daunting. It's the magic of love that can conquer all obstacles. She has seen me planning things for my child day and night and how I was so much into learning new skills and adapting to new situations so that I can help my son to adapt to the new situation as well. I used to spend hours talking to therapists to learn skills, I used to watch various videos of therapies to meet needs of autistic children.

Theme 4: Advocacy for Change

A prominent thread woven throughout the mother's narrative was her fervent advocacy for change in the system. From calling for greater inclusivity in education to championing societal acceptance and understanding of autism, she articulated a passionate desire to effect positive change for her child and others like him. Her narrative served as a powerful call to action, urging stakeholders to prioritise the needs of autistic individuals and their families in policy, practice, and public discourse.

> My journey with my son has ignited a fire within me, a burning passion to break down barriers and pave the way for a more inclusive world. Every word I speak is a plea for change, for a society that embraces neurodiversity with open arms. I advocate for my son and all those who walk a similar path, demanding better

> support, understanding, and opportunities. My voice may tremble at times, but my resolve remains unwavering. I won't rest until every door is open, every mind enlightened, and every heart filled with compassion for autism. This is not just my battle; it's a collective call to arms for a world where every individual is valued and celebrated for who they are.

Theme 5: Hope and Resilience

Despite the myriad challenges encountered during the pandemic, the mother's narrative was imbued with a sense of hope and resilience. She expressed optimism about her child's potential for growth and development, buoyed by the unwavering support of her family and community. Her narrative served as a poignant reminder of the indomitable spirit of parents and caregivers navigating the complex terrain of autism with courage, compassion, and unwavering determination.

> In the darkest of times, I find my strength in the flicker of hope that dances within my heart. Despite the storms we've weathered, I believe in a future where my child thrives, where his laughter echoes through the halls of possibility. With each sunrise, I am reminded of the resilience that resides within us, a beacon guiding us through the labyrinth of challenges. Surrounded by the love of family and the warmth of our community, I am filled with gratitude for the journey we walk together. Autism may present hurdles, but it also unveils hidden strengths and boundless possibilities. As we journey forward, hand in hand, I embrace the promise of tomorrow with unwavering faith and unyielding hope.

Theme 6: New Found Relationship

The theme "new found relationship" encapsulates the profound shift in the mother–child chemistry that emerged from a fresh perspective as a result of the extended time spent together during the pandemic. The mother's reflections suggest that the pandemic facilitated a deeper emotional connection. This was achieved through increased interaction and the necessity of creating new routines and activities that both mother and child could engage in. The shared experiences and joint problem-solving fostered a sense of partnership and mutual understanding.

> The pandemic, despite all its challenges, brought an unexpected positive change in our relationship. With the lockdown, we spent more time together than ever before. Initially, it was overwhelming for both of us, but over time, I started understanding my child's needs and emotions on a much deeper level. We developed new routines and activities that we both enjoyed, and this created a stronger bond between us. I feel more connected to my child now, and this newfound relationship has given me more insight and patience. It's like we've created our own way of communicating and understanding each other, something we didn't have before the lockdown.

Discussion

Autism or ASD is a "neurodevelopmental disorder". The worldwide prevalence of ASD is about 1 in 59 children and in India, it is estimated to be 1 in 100 children aged 2–9 years (Arora et al., 2018). However, there continues to be a deficit of trained therapists to address these children (Mahapatra et al., 2019). Moreover, parents may observe deviations in their child's growth and development when compared to peers within their social circles, family, and friends. These observations often become more pronounced when the child enters preschool. Typically, signs of developmental differences can be detected around the age of three. Formal assessments and diagnostic testing are often initiated upon recommendation from healthcare clinics or educational institutions (Constantino et al., 2020; Keehn et al., 2020; van 't Hof et al., 2021).

The study focused on uncovering both their initial concerns and subsequent coping mechanisms during the COVID-19 pandemic lockdown. Initially, the mother expressed widespread apprehension regarding the abrupt shift in routines and the cessation of therapeutic interventions, recognising the potential for developmental regression and heightened behavioural challenges. These worries mirrored established research emphasising the importance of therapies in addressing social and behavioural deficits in individuals with autism (DeFilippis & Wagner, 2016; Landa, 2007). Moreover, concerns extended to the mother's ability to provide adequate support and education to her son, highlighting the interconnectedness of her wellbeing and the child's outcomes (Hall, 2012; Twoy et al., 2007; Wodehouse & McGill, 2009). This underscores the need for tailored interventions and ongoing support for families navigating the complexities of autism during crises such as the pandemic.

Thus, one can conclude that as the lockdown persisted, families encountered diverse challenges, with many exacerbated by pre-existing difficulties common in autism. These challenges can significantly test the emotional resilience of parents, who had to manage children without any prior training or support. The abrupt disruption of routine and social isolation required parents to demonstrate adaptive resilience by developing new routines and strategies to cope with these changes. Moreover, the situation underscored the importance of resilience, as parents had to rely more on their resources and skills rather than external support systems. This period of prolonged adversity highlighted the persistence and growth of parents as they continuously adapted and learned to better support their children amidst the ongoing challenges. Parents' efforts to establish adapted routines and create conducive home environments varied in effectiveness, highlighting the importance of personalised support and guidance for families (Factor et al., 2016; Souders et al., 2009).

Conclusion

The present case study focused experiences of a mother of a child who was diagnosed with ASD at the age of 4, with marked differences in terms of his delayed speech, social interaction, hyperactivity, and fine motor skills. The present study highlights the phenomenon of neuro-divergence in the context of the caregiver's (mother) experience during the COVID-19 pandemic. The major themes that emerged include 'resilience in adversity', 'struggles with social isolation', 'adaptation and creativity', 'advocacy for change', and 'hope and resilience'. It was also observed that the mother expressed a sense of a newfound relationship established between the mother and the child with other positive elements consisting of finding an interest in the area of music by the child, with more autonomous expression and functioning being inculcated within the child, as a consequence of the pandemic. On the other hand, the lack of social interaction, community support, and a sense of loneliness during the challenging circumstances of the pandemic served as a bane to the overall experience of the mother.

Implications

This case study underscores the importance of resilience and adaptability in the face of challenges. Mothers of autistic children can draw inspiration from the example set by the mother in this study, recognising that even during unprecedented times like the COVID-19 pandemic, learning new skills and adapting to changing circumstances can significantly benefit their child's development and education. The mother's efforts to acquire new skills during the pandemic demonstrate the value of continuous learning and proactive problem-solving. Mothers of autistic children are encouraged to seek out resources, training, and support networks that can equip them with strategies and tools to better support their child's unique needs.

The importance of support systems, whether through formal educational resources, online communities, or local support groups, is well established by the literature. Building a network of support can provide emotional assistance, practical advice, and a sense of community, helping mothers feel less isolated in their caregiving journey. This case also illustrates the powerful role that mothers can play as advocates for their children. By being informed, proactive, and resilient, mothers can better navigate educational and healthcare systems, ensuring their children receive the necessary support and accommodations. Empowerment through knowledge and advocacy can lead to improved outcomes for their children.

Lastly, this study serves as a source of hope and inspiration. The mother's unwavering commitment and successful efforts to support her child's growth despite significant challenges offer a message of hope. The findings of the present study can be instrumental in developing effective interventions, policies, and societal changes that help enhance the wellbeing and opportunities for both neurodivergent individuals and their caregivers.

Limitations

This analysis is based on a single case, which limits the generalisability of the findings. The experiences and strategies of one mother may not be representative of all mothers of autistic children, given the diversity in individual circumstances, resources, and support systems. The insights and observations are inherently subjective, influenced by the author's perspective and the mother's account. This subjectivity can affect the objectivity and broader applicability of the conclusions drawn.

The case study provides a snapshot of the mother's experiences during a specific period, particularly the COVID-19 pandemic. It lacks longitudinal insights that could reveal how her strategies and the child's development evolve over a more extended period. Also, the insights from the father have not been considered in the present case study. The mother's ability to learn new skills and support her child during the pandemic may have been influenced by the availability of resources such as internet access, financial stability, and educational materials, which might not be accessible to all mothers in similar situations. While the study highlights the mother's resilience, it does not deeply explore the psychological impact of her dual challenges on her mental health and wellbeing, which is crucial for understanding the full scope of her experience.

Funding

This research received no external funding.

Declaration of Conflicting Interests

The author(s) declared no potential conflicts of interest concerning the research, authorship, and/or publication of this article.

References

Agazzi, H., Adams, C., Ferron, E., Ferron, J., Shaffer-Hudkins, E., & Salloum, A. (2019). Trauma-informed behavioral parenting for early intervention. *Journal of Child and Family Studies*, *28*, 2172–2186.

Armstrong, T. (2015). The myth of the normal brain: Embracing neurodiversity. *American Medical Association Journal of Ethics*, *17*(4), 348–352.

Arora, N. K., Nair, M. K. C., Gulati, S., Deshmukh, V., Mohapatra, A., Mishra, D., ... & Vajaratkar, V. (2018). Neurodevelopmental disorders in children aged 2–9 years: Population-based burden estimates across five regions in India. *PLoS Medicine*, *15*(7), e1002615.

Blacher, J., & Christensen, L. (2011). Sowing the seeds of the autism field: Leo Kanner (1943). *Intellectual and Developmental Disabilities*, *49*(3), 172–191.

Blume, H. (1998). Neurodiversity: On the neurological underpinnings of geekdom. *The Atlantic*, *30*.

Botha, M., Chapman, R., Giwa Onaiwu, M., Kapp, S. K., Stannard Ashley, A., & Walker, N. (2024). The neurodiversity concept was developed collectively: An overdue correction on the origins of neurodiversity theory. *Autism*, *28*(6), 1591–1594.

Bottema-Beutel, K., Kapp, S. K., Lester, J. N., Sasson, N. J., & Hand, B. N. (2021). Avoiding ableist language: Suggestions for autism researchers. *Autism in Adulthood*.

Braun, V., & Clarke, V. (2006). Using thematic analysis in psychology. *Qualitative Research in Psychology, 3*, 77–101.

Buijsman, R., Begeer, S., & Scheeren, A. M. (2023). 'Autistic person' or 'person with autism'? Person-first language preference in Dutch adults with autism and parents. *Autism, 27*(3), 788–795.

Bury, S. M., Jellett, R., Spoor, J. R., & Hedley, D. (2023). "It defines who I am" or "It's something I have": What language do [autistic] Australian adults [on the autism spectrum] prefer?. *Journal of Autism and Developmental Disorders, 53*(2), 677–687.

Cascio, M. A. (2015). Cross-cultural autism studies, neurodiversity, and conceptualizations of autism. *Culture, Medicine, and Psychiatry, 39*, 207–212.

Chapman, R. (2019a). Neurodiversity theory and its discontents: Autism, schizophrenia, and the social model of disability. *The Bloomsbury Companion to Philosophy of Psychiatry, 371*.

Chapman, R. (2019b). Autism as a form of life: Wittgenstein and the psychological coherence of autism. *Metaphilosophy, 50*(4), 421–440.

Charlton, J. I. (1998). *Nothing About Us Without Us: Disability Oppression and Empowerment*. University of California Press.

Chown, N., & Beavan, N. (2012). Intellectually capable but socially excluded? A review of the literature and research on students with autism in further education. *Journal of Further and Higher Education, 36*(4), 477–493.

Cleary, M., West, S., & Mclean, L. (2023). From 'refrigerator mothers' to empowered advocates: The evolution of the autism parent. *Issues in Mental Health Nursing, 44*(1), 64–70.

Cohmer, S. (2014). Early infantile autism and the refrigerator mother theory (1943-1970). *Embryo Project Encyclopedia*.

Constantino, J. N., Abbacchi, A. M., Saulnier, C., Klaiman, C., Mandell, D. S., Zhang, Y., ... & Geschwind, D. H. (2020). Timing of the diagnosis of autism in African American children. *Pediatrics, 146*(3).

DeFilippis M., & Wagner K. D. (2016). Treatment of autism spectrum disorder in children and adolescents. *Psychopharmacology Bulletin*, 46(2), 18–41. www.ncbi.nlm.nih.gov/pubmed/27738378

Doyle, N., Hough, L., Thorne, K., & Banfield, T. (2022). Neurodiversity. In *Challenging Bias in Forensic Psychological Assessment and Testing* (pp. 329–357). Routledge.

Estes, A., Munson, J., Dawson, G., Koehler, E., Zhou, X. H., & Abbott, R. (2009). Parenting stress and psychological functioning among mothers of preschool children with autism and developmental delay. *Autism, 13*(4), 375–387.

Factor, R. S., Condy, E. E., Farley, J. P., & Scarpa, A. (2016). Brief report: Insistence on sameness, anxiety, and social motivation in children with autism spectrum disorder. *Journal of Autism and Developmental Disorders, 46*, 2548–2554.

Hall, H. R. (2012). Families of children with autism: Behaviors of children, community support and coping. *Issues in Comprehensive Pediatric Nursing, 35*(2), 111–132. https://doi.org/10.3109/01460862.2012.678263

Hassenfeldt, T. A., Lorenzi, J., & Scarpa, A. (2015). A review of parent training in child interventions: applications to cognitive–behavioral therapy for children with high-functioning autism. *Review Journal of Autism and Developmental Disorders, 2*, 79–90.

Hayes, S. A., & Watson, S. L. (2013). The impact of parenting stress: A meta-analysis of studies comparing the experience of parenting stress in parents of children with and without autism spectrum disorder. *Journal of Autism and Developmental Disorders, 43*, 629–642.

Hughes, J. M. (2016). Increasing neurodiversity in disability and social justice advocacy groups. *Autistic Self Advocacy Network.*

Jansen, D. E., Carai, S., Scott, E., Butu, C., Pop, I., Park, M., ... & Wolfe, I. (2022). COVID-19 has exposed the need for health system assessments to be more child health-sensitive. *Journal of Global Health, 12.*

Jurgens, A. (2021). Re-conceptualizing the role of stimuli: An enactive, ecological explanation of spontaneous-response tasks. *Phenomenology and the Cognitive Sciences, 20*(5), 915–934.

Kanner, L. (1943). *Intellectual and Developmental Disabilities, 49*(3), 172–191.

Kapp, S. (2019). How social deficit models exacerbate the medical model: Autism as case in point. *Autism Policy & Practice, 2*(1), 3–28.

Kapp, S. K. (2020). *Autistic Community and the Neurodiversity Movement: Stories from the Frontline* (p. 330). Springer Nature.

Karmakar, S. N. (2023). A prospective study of socioeconomic status by modified Kuppuswamy scale in cases of suicidal deaths: An autopsy based analysis. *Journal of Indian Academy of Forensic Medicine, 45*(3), 211–215.

Keehn, R. M. N., Ciccarelli, M., Szczepaniak, D., Tomlin, A., Lock, T., & Swigonski, N. (1 August 2020). A statewide tiered system for screening and diagnosis of autism spectrum disorder. *Pediatrics, 146*, 20193876. https://doi.org/10.1542/peds.2019-3876

Kenny, L., Hattersley, C., Molins, B., Buckley, C., Povey, C., & Pellicano, E. (2016). Which terms should be used to describe autism? Perspectives from the UK autism community. *Autism, 20*(4), 442–462.

Kotsopoulou, A., Papadaki, E., Florou, I., Troupou, A., Kolosioni, D., Georgiou, A., ... & Koumanioti, E. (2021). Parents of children with autistic spectrum disorder (ASD) as co-therapists: The therapists' view. *Psychology, 11*(2), 44–55.

Lai, M. C., & Baron-Cohen, S. (2015). Identifying the lost generation of adults with autism spectrum conditions. *The Lancet Psychiatry, 2*(11), 1013–1027.

Landa, R. (2007). Early communication development and intervention for children with autism. *Mental Retardation and Developmental Disabilities Research Reviews, 13*(1), 16–25.

Langan, M. (2011). Parental voices and controversies in autism. *Disability & Society, 26*(2), 193–205.

Leadbitter, K., Buckle, K. L., Ellis, C., & Dekker, M. (2021). Autistic self-advocacy and the neurodiversity movement: Implications for autism early intervention research and practice. *Frontiers in Psychology, 12*, 635690.

Levitt, J. (2017). *Exploring how the Social Model of Disability Can be Re-Invigorated: In Response to.*

Mahapatra, P., Pati, S., Sinha, R., Chauhan, A. S., Nanda, R. R., & Nallala, S. (2019). Parental care-seeking pathway and challenges for autistic spectrum disorders children: A mixed method study from Bhubaneswar, Odisha. *Indian Journal of Psychiatry, 61*(1), 37–44.

Oliver, M. (1983). *Social Work with Disabled People*. Macmillan.

Oliver, M. (2013). The social model of disability: Thirty years on. *Disability & Society, 28*(7), 1024–1026.

Olkin, R. (2002). Could you hold the door for me? Including disability in diversity. *Cultural Diversity and Ethnic Minority Psychology, 8*, 130–137.

Pellicano, E., & den Houting, J. (2022). Annual research review: Shifting from 'normal science' to neurodiversity in autism science. *Journal of Child Psychology and Psychiatry, 63*(4), 381–396.

Pellicano, E., & Stears, M. (2020). The hidden inequalities of COVID-19. *Autism, 24*(6), 1309–1310.

Prata, J., Lawson, W., & Coelho, R. (2018). Parent training for parents of children on the autism spectrum: a review. *Health, 5*(3), 1–8.

Pripas-Kapit, S. (2020). Historicizing Jim Sinclair's "Don't mourn for us": A cultural and intellectual history of neurodiversity's first manifesto. In *Autistic Community and the Neurodiversity Movement: Stories from the Frontline*, 23–39.

Rajaraman, K., & Mundkur, N. (2021). Parent-mediated training for children with autism spectrum disorder in India. *Indian Pediatrics, 58*(7), 692–692.

Rodriguez, G., Hartley, S. L., & Bolt, D. (2019). Transactional relations between parenting stress and child autism symptoms and behavior problems. *Journal of Autism and Developmental Disorders, 49*, 1887–1898.

Sheffer, E. (2018). *Asperger's Children: The Origins of Autism in Nazi Vienna*. WW Norton & Company.

Silberman, S. (2017). Neurodiversity rewires conventional thinking about brains. In *Beginning with Disability* (pp. 51–52). Routledge.

Sinclair, J. (1999). *Don't Mourn for Us*. Autistic Rights Movement UK.

Singer, H. S., Giuliano, J. D., Hansen, B. H., Hallett, J. J., Laurino, J. P., Benson, M., & Kiessling, L. S. (1998). Antibodies against human putamen in children with Tourette syndrome. *Neurology, 50*(6), 1618–1624.

Singer, J. (1999). Why can't you be normal for once in your life? From a problem with no name to the emergence of a new category of difference. *Disability Discourse,* 59–67.

Smail, D. (2005). *Power, Interest and Psychology: Elements of a Social Materialist Understanding of Distress*. PCCS Books.

Souders, M. C., Mason, T. B., Valladares, O., Bucan, M., Levy, S. E., Mandell, D. S., & Pinto-Martin, J. (2009). Sleep behaviors and sleep quality in children with autism spectrum disorders. *Sleep*, 32(12), 1566–1578. https://doi.org/10.1093/sleep/32.12.1566

Stanton-Chapman, T. L., & Schmidt, E. L. (2019). In search of equivalent social participation: What do caregivers of children with disabilities desire regarding inclusive recreational facilities and playgrounds?. *Journal of International Special Needs Education, 22*(2), 66–76.

Swanke, J., Zeman, L. D., & Doktor, J. (2009). Discontent and activism among mothers who blog while raising children with autism spectrum disorders. *Journal of the Motherhood Initiative for Research and Community Involvement.*

Taboas, A., Doepke, K., & Zimmerman, C. (2023). Preferences for identity-first versus person-first language in a US sample of autism stakeholders. *Autism, 27*(2), 565–570.

Tokatly Latzer, I., Leitner, Y., & Karnieli-Miller, O. (2021). Core experiences of parents of children with autism during the COVID-19 pandemic lockdown. *Autism, 25*(4), 1047–1059.

Twoy, R., Connolly, P. M., & Novak, J. M. (2007). Coping strategies used by parents of children with autism. *Journal of the American Association of Nurse Practitioners, 19*(5), 251–260.

van 't Hof, M., Tisseur, C., van Berckelear-Onnes, I., van Nieuwenhuyzen, A., Daniels, A. M., Deen, M., … & Ester, W. A. (1 May 2021). Age at autism spectrum disorder diagnosis: A systematic review and metaanalysis from 2012 to 2019. *Autism, 25*, 862–873. https://doi.org/10.1177/1362361320971107

Vilaseca, R., Ferrer, F., & Guardia Olmos, J. (2014). Gender differences in positive perceptions, anxiety, and depression among mothers and fathers of children with intellectual disabilities: a logistic regression analysis. *Quality & Quantity, 48*, 2241–2253.

Vivanti, G. (2020). Ask the editor: What is the most appropriate way to talk about individuals with a diagnosis of autism?. *Journal of Autism and Developmental Disorders*, *50*(2), 691–693.

Watts, G. (2014). Lorna wing. *The Lancet*, *384*(9944), 658.

Wodehouse, G., & McGill, P. (2009). Support for family carers of children and young people with developmental disabilities and challenging behaviour: what stops it being helpful? *Journal of Intellectual Disability Research*, *53*(7), 644–653. https://doi.org/10.1111/j.1365-2788.2009.01163.x

Woods, R. (2017). Exploring how the social model of disability can be re-invigorated for autism: in response to Jonathan Levitt. *Disability & Society*, *32*(7), 1090–1095.

Appendix (Interview Schedule)

Q1. Can you share when your child was diagnosed with autism? How did you feel when you received the diagnosis?

Q2. Can you describe a typical day in your life before the COVID-19 pandemic? How did you manage your child's daily routines and activities?

Q3. How did the COVID-19 pandemic initially affect your daily life and routines? What were the immediate challenges you faced when the pandemic began?

Q4. What changes did you have to make to your child's routine and your caregiving practices during the pandemic? How did you adapt to these changes?

Q5. How did your access to support systems change during the pandemic? Were there any new sources of support that emerged during this time?

Q6. How did the stress of the pandemic and caring for an autistic child affect your mental and emotional wellbeing? What coping mechanisms or strategies did you find helpful during this time?

Q7. How did you manage your child's education and learning needs during the pandemic? What new skills or knowledge did you acquire to support your child's learning?

Q8. What have you learned about yourself and your child through the experiences of the pandemic?
Are there any new perspectives or insights that you have gained?

Q9. Is there anything else you would like to share about your experiences during the pandemic?
Do you have any questions or final thoughts?

Follow-up questions were asked as and when required.

9 Pandemic and Pride

Shame, Guilt, and Self-Esteem in LGBTQIA+ and Heterosexual Individuals

A. A. S. Azam, Rudra Vijhani, Ketoki Mazumdar, and Fouzia A. Shaikh

Introduction

India has always had a rich and varied past and culture that embraces and celebrates the 'existence'. India has rich traditions that reference the ideals of spreading love, coexistence, and compassionate living. The mediaeval temples of Khajuraho in Madhya Pradesh, which date back to the 12th century and are well-known for their blatantly sensual carvings that also show sexual fluidity, are amazing examples of this inclusivity. Shakuntala Devi's (1977) publication of *The World of Homosexuals*, the country's first research on homosexuality, was a pivotal point in the acceptance of LGBTQIA+ concerns. One worldwide poll by Institut Public de Sondage d'OpinionSecteur (IPSOS), indicates that 17% of Indians do not identify as heterosexual. Of this group, 9% identify as bisexual, 3% as lesbian, gay, or homosexual, 1% identify as asexual, 2% as pansexual or omnisexual, and 2% as belonging to other identities (IPSOS, 2021).

Identity and social acceptance related social, cognitive, and emotional challenges have been well documented in a recent Indian study by Mohan (2022) which noted stigma-driven shame and guilt as significant causes of chronic stress, homophobia along with other mental health disorders and physical health ailments in the LGBTQIA+ communities. Self-esteem or evaluations of oneself is an inherent cognitive consequence of experiences of shame and guilt. Shame and guilt are self-conscious emotions experienced when one evaluates abilities and performance in designated social roles and responsibilities (Choi, 2024). Choi (2024) further offered a clear distinction between the two emotions – shame as more associated with stable, rigid, and negative evaluations of self while guilt as more associated with adaptive and flexible evaluations of personal abilities and attributes. While both shame and guilt are predominantly negative experiences, evidence suggests that those sexual minorities with shame-proneness, are more vulnerable to mental health problems, substance abuse, sexual disorders, and interpersonal problems in comparison to their guilt-prone counterparts (Kidd et al., 2018;Rapinda et al., 2021).

According to Mohan's (2022) overview of sexual minority groups in India, LGBTQIA+ is an umbrella term comprising people identifying as Lesbian, Gay, Bisexual, Transgender, Queer, and over 60 other genders. Lesbian is a woman who has a romantic or sexual orientation towards other women, Gay refers to men who

DOI: 10.4324/9781003517313-10

have a romantic or sexual orientation towards other men, Bisexual is a person who has a romantic or sexual orientation towards both men and women, Transgender is a person whose gender identity is different from the gender they were assigned at birth, Queer is a term used by individuals who are still unsure about their identity and are in process of figuring it out (Mohan, 2022).

Even though the COVID-19-related social–emotional struggles of sexual minority groups worldwide were prominent, there is relatively less research evidence about the struggles and challenges faced by them.

For LGBTQIA+ individuals, the pandemic heightened several psychosocial stress factors, revealing vulnerabilities that extend beyond the general population's experience for example, Approximately, 28% of LGBTQIA+ college students were concerned about accessing care during the pandemic due to their identity, with 40% reporting unmet mental health needs, and a quarter worried about physical safety or financial security, with some forced to return to the closet (Gonzales et al., 2023). Among younger students, Hispanic/Latinx students, and students from unsupportive homes or colleges, a few of these negative effects were more common. LGBTQIA+ people are known to be at risk for comorbid psycho-social stress factors, which include mood disorders, complex trauma, chronic stress, generalised anxiety and distress, and adjustment disorders (Li et al., 2023). People who experience social stigma and constraints, such as members of the LGBTQIA+ community, have particular worries that are often disregarded and kept silent, even though the general public is susceptible to dread, and anxiety related to pandemics (Bannerjee & Nair, 2020). During the pandemic, approximately half of the research study participants experienced severe or extremely severe depression, an unusually high for the population (Das & Govindappa, 2023). Increased symptoms of anxiety and despair were also linked to symptoms of post-traumatic stress disorder (PTSD), loneliness, concerns about the severity of COVID-19, and associated grieving. Relationship problems, thoughts of suicide, substance misuse, and disordered eating patterns were also some of the prominent problems of the sexual minority group members (Datta & Mukherjee, 2023). Compared to heterosexuals, sexual minorities are therefore more likely to have several subsequent disorders that are linked to serious COVID-19–related illnesses. The discriminatory and stigmatising experiences in healthcare (both mental and physical) access and provider ignorance can be considered as the salient causes of these heightened psychological and behavioural hazards, including shame and guilt, for the LGBTQIA+ community (Krause, 2021).

Literature accounts for familial influences (Peters et al., 2019), traumatic experiences, self-reported mental and physical health (Scheer et al., 2020), interpersonal stigma such as past-year family rejection and childhood bullying (Pachankis & Hatzenbuehler, 2024) as some of the factors seen playing a role in shame and guilt in the sexual minorities.

While there is a plethora of studies highlighting the causes and consequences of social stigma in LGBTQIA+ communities, there are fewer studies that specifically examine shame and guilt-related self-perceptions in these social groups in the Indian context. Mishra (2020), in an ethnographic study, examined the self-perceptions of a group of participants from the gay community and found that while guilt-related perceptions of the self, continued to have internal causality, the guilt responses reported by the participants were predominantly heteronormative (Mishra, 2020). Studies by Breakwell (2020) and Breakwell and Jaspal (2022) revealed a strong connection between how perception of self and identity further define one's experience of internal shame. However, sparse studies about shame and guilt experiences of LGBTQIA+ communities have been conducted in India, especially COVID-19 experiences that could determine whether these experiences are more heteronormative or more influenced by their individualistic evaluations of self traits and gender identity. The study was therefore undertaken to get an empirical understanding of shame, guilt, and self-esteem evaluations of urban Indian sexual minorities and heterosexual groups, stemming from their experiences during the COVID-19 period.

There has been a positive change in acceptance over the last couple of years, with South Africa and India recording the highest increases (Dyvik, 2024). This suggests that India is progressing towards greater acceptance of LGBTQIA+ individuals, despite shame and guilt still being predominantly heteronormative in the contemporary homosexual communities in India (Mishra, 2020). The emerging acceptance of sexual minority sections of Indian society can be considered an indicator of improved perceptions of self and lesser lived experiences related to guilt and shame across the gender spectrum. Nonetheless on account of the scarcity of Indian research studies addressing guilt, shame, and self-perceptions in LGBTQIA+ individuals alongside their heterosexual counterparts since COVID-19, the present study was undertaken.

Significance of the Study

The current paper explored the differences felt in self-esteem along with shame and guilt amongst heterosexual men and women and the LGBTQIA+ community. With the growing acceptance of the LGBTQIA+ community, it was essential to address the stigmas related to the community, discrimination, and marginalisation faced by them to foster greater acceptance and support within society and individuals themselves. Discrimination and social stigma-oriented internalised shame were found to increase anxiety and depression levels in the LGBTQIA+ community, especially among LGBTQIA+ women (Cabral & Pinto, 2023). LGBTQ+ individuals were found to be victims of health vulnerabilities due to social and political inequalities (Mink et al., 2014). Studies suggested that cisgender individuals were more prone to poor health outcomes as COVID-19 impacted them due to the disparities and inequities prevalent during the pandemic (Kline, 2020). As mental health services alongside other common and crucial healthcare services faced massive interruptions in terms of provision and access during the pandemic years, it became imperative to address the unheard voices related to self and society in the marginalised social and sexual minority groups of India.

Objectives

1 To examine the interplay of the relationship between shame, guilt, and self-esteem
2 To compare the two groups, the LGBTQIA+ community and the heterosexual men and women on shame, guilt, and self-esteem.

Method

Hypotheses

H_1: There will be a significant difference between shame and guilt between heterosexual men and women and the LGBTQIA+ community.
H_2: There will be a significant difference in self-esteem between heterosexual men and women and the LGBTQIA+ community.
H_3: There will be a significant negative relationship between shame, guilt, and self-esteem across both groups.

Sample

A combination of convenience sampling and snowball sampling, both non-probability sampling techniques, was employed to recruit participants from a population that is difficult to access due to pervasive social stigmas associated with non-normative gender identities. These methods allowed the researchers to effectively reach individuals within the LGBTQIA+ community, leveraging existing social networks to identify additional participants who might otherwise remain hidden due to fear of discrimination or social exclusion. A total of 130 Individuals participated, 50% being heterosexual men and women (n = 65) and 50% being LGBTQIA+ (n = 65). Of the LGBTQIA+ individuals' the majority of the representation was bisexual (n = 10), gay (n = 5), lesbian (n = 3), asexual (n = 2), and others. The age range of the participants was 17–42 years.

Research Design

The current study employed a comparative and cross-sectional research design to examine the relationship between shame, guilt, and self-esteem, as well as to compare the LGBTQIA+ community and heterosexual men and women on these variables.

Inclusion and Exclusion Criteria

Measures

Demographics

Upon checking the inclusion and exclusion criteria mentioned in Table 9.1, the demographics, such as age, residential status, whether from the LGBTQIA+

Table 9.1 Inclusion and exclusion criteria

Inclusion criteria	*Exclusion criteria*
Should be above 17 and below 42 years	Gender-fluid or gender non-conforming participants
Should be of Indian nationality and residing in India at the time of participation	Participants reportedly lived outside India at the time of the survey
Individuals who chose one clear gender identity option from amongst the given options in the demographic form	Individuals who did not choose any one of the gender identity options in the demographic form

community, gender preference (if applicable), and family type, play a crucial role in understanding the social and psychological dynamics of individuals. Participants were asked to fill out the informed consent in which participants were apprised of the purpose of the study and were also assured of the confidentiality of their responses.

Guilt and Shame-8 Questionnaire

The Guilt and Shame-8 Questionnaire (Hoppen et al., 2022) was used and unidimensional shame and guilt scores were computed for each participant. On a non-clinical sample, Cronbach's alpha was 0.83. Internal consistencies were acceptable for the guilt factor 0.74, and for the shame factor was 0.82. It uses a 5-point response format with the response option (0) 'never', (1) 'once or twice', (2) 'three to four times', and (3) 'daily'. The participants were asked to indicate how frequently they had experienced each item in the past 4 weeks. The levels of shame and guilt were categorised as low when the total score was below 6, average when the total score ranged between 7 and 11, and high when the total score exceeded 12. The scoring value ranged from 0 to 32.

Rosenberg Self-Esteem Scale (RSES)

The RSES is a 10-item unidimensional scale developed by Rosenberg which was designed to assess self-esteem in terms of overall self-worth by assessing both positive and negative thoughts about oneself (Rosenberg, 1965). The response pattern adopted a 4-point Likert scale, ranging from 'strongly agree' to 'strongly disagree'. A study by Monteiro et al. (2021) revealed strong predictive validity, internal consistency, and test-retest reliability for the RSES. The internal consistency coefficient for the test was found to be 0.90 (Monteiro et al., 2021). Scores ranged from 0 to 40 and were categorised into three levels: low self-esteem was below 25, average self-esteem was between 26 and 30, and high self-esteem was 31 and above.

Procedure

The standardised questionnaires along with demographic and informed consent forms were circulated through online platforms. The snowball sampling method helped the researchers to get in touch with adults and college goers from various institutions. Participants were also encouraged to reach out to the researcher, through e-mail or feasible social media (WhatsApp), in case of any doubt, or query related to any statement in the form and also if they further wanted to know their scores on the different tests. All the participants who approached the researcher(s) personally through email and feasible social media (WhatsApp) were further helped with their queries and concerns, especially regarding survey interpretation and results.

Statistical Analysis

The data were initially exported to Microsoft Excel, where alphabetical values were coded into numeric values for processing in JAMOVI 2.3.28 and IBM SPSS Statistics version 20. Statistical analysis techniques such as the Shapiro–Wilk test for normality, skewness and kurtosis assessments, descriptive statistics, Kendall Tau's B, and its scatter plots. Since the Shapiro–Wilk test for normality revealed deviation of the data from normality, the non-parametric Brunner–Munzel test was performed to compare self-esteem and shame-guilt scores between heterosexual and LGBTQIA+ groups

Results

Table 9.2 shows the descriptive statistics based on self-reported gender identity. For the LGBTQIA+ community, shame-guilt and self-esteem were found to be in the average range. Shame-guilt and self-esteem scores for heterosexual group members were also found to be in the average range.

Table 9.3 shows that all of the variables were reported to be asymptotic. There were no statistically significant differences ($p = 0.05$) obtained between the LGBTQIA+ community and heterosexual individuals.

Table 9.2 Descriptive statistics of shame-guilt and self-esteem scores

Variable	*Gender identity*	*n*	*Mean*	*SD*
Shame and guilt	LGBTQIA+	65	9.66	7.38
	Heterosexual	65	9.74	6.21
Self-esteem	LGBTQIA+	65	26.7	5.92
	Heterosexual	65	28.1	5.18

Table 9.3 Brunner–Munzel test

		Statistic	*df*	*p*
Self-esteem	Asymptotic	1.697	125	0.092
Shame and guilt	Asymptotic	0.458	122	0.647

$p > 0.05$

Table 9.4 Kendall Tau's B correlation between shame-guilt and self-esteem

Variables	*Self-esteem*
Shame and guilt	-0.315*

$^{*}p < 0.001$

Table 9.4 depicts a negative and statistically significant correlation between shame-guilt and self-esteem scores which indicated that the higher the level of shame-guilt, the lower the participants' self-esteem and vice-versa.

Discussion

The present study provided an overview of the relationship between guilt, shame, and self-esteem ratings of LGBTQIA+ and heterosexual participants in the study. The descriptive statistics (Table 9.2) showed that shame and guilt were experienced similarly by LGBTQIA+ and heterosexual people. Also, their scores were found to be in the average range. This finding, however, was not in accordance with previous recent literature which claimed that shame and guilt experiences among sexual minorities were particularly higher in situations of adversity (e.g., COVID-19) that are profoundly characterised by economic hardships and health inequities (Gil et al., 2021; Mink et al., 2014). The above-average shame-guilt scores obtained in the present study (Table 9.1) were suggestive that despite the difficulties encountered by the LGBTQIA+ participants in the study, during COVID-19 years, other individualistic protective factors like identity integration and religious orientation were prevalent as their vital resources for controlling these self-related emotions and attributions (Anderson & Koc, 2020).

The present study tested the alternative hypothesis that shame, guilt, and self-esteem would significantly differ between heterosexual and LGBTQIA+ groups. However, as indicated by Table 9.3, no statistically significant mean difference was found in the shame-guilt scores between the two groups, leading to the rejection of the alternative hypothesis. This finding is particularly notable, as limited recent research (Cabral & Pinto, 2023) was found to be specifically focused on comparing shame-guilt responses between homosexual and heterosexual individuals in situations of adversity. Thus, this result provided a unique contribution to the literature, emphasising the need for further exploration in this area, where empirical studies remain sparse. This finding indicated that the intensity of these self-conscious emotions was not greater in LGBTQIA+ individuals compared to heterosexual individuals. The findings possibly indicate that shame-guilt perceptions are not solely determined by one's gender identity or perceived sexual orientation. Rather, these emotional experiences may also be influenced by a range of cultural and protective factors (Luthar et al., 2015) that were beyond the scope of this study. Consequently, the present study findings hinted towards the complexity of these self-defining emotions and addressed the need for future research to examine additional variables that may shape self-conscious feelings across different sexual minority and heterosexual groups. One of the reasons behind similar levels of reported shame, guilt and self-esteem scores could be attributed to not further classifying the two sample groups (i.e., LGBTQIA+ and homosexual) into their constituent gender groups. For instance, Ovesen (2023) examined the experiences of shame and guilt amongst LGBTQIA+ community members and found that queer and lesbian participants expressed shame due to lack of social support and retaliatory response to violence and abuse in past relationships. The present study findings also contradicted previous research evidence in which LGBTQIA+ individuals reported higher levels of shame experience in comparison to their heterosexual counterparts (Cabral & Pinto, 2023). This could be due to the non-inclusion of potentially protective factors like identity resilience, self-efficacy (Breakwell, 2020), and social support from family, friends, and peers (Stotzer et al., 2014) which are known to influence self-esteem across diverse gender orientations (Cabral & Pinto, 2023).

This study also yielded a negative statistically significant correlation of self-esteem with shame and guilt perception as presented in Table 9.4 and Figure 9.1.

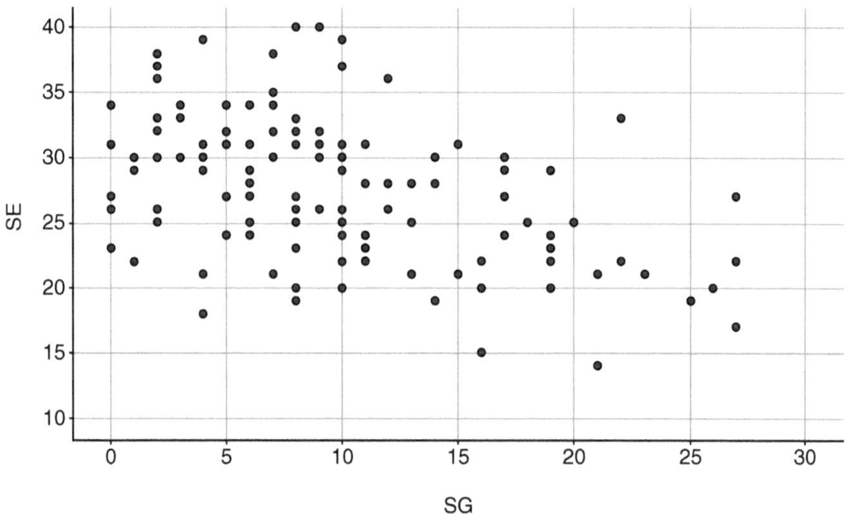

Figure 9.1 Kendall Tau's B scatterplot for self-esteem and shame-guilt.

This finding aligned with that of Cabral and Pinto (2023) which indicated that higher shame scores were correlated with low-esteem scores. Guilt, shame, and self-esteem correlations were also accompanied by large effect sizes in earlier studies (Budiarto & Helmi, 2021). The present study therefore continued to consolidate the adverse effects of shame-guilt perceptions on self-worth evaluations across the entire gender spectrum. The inverse association between both variables can be considered as the result of latent deep-rooted discriminatory experiences like denial of access to health care, education, and other forms of social support on grounds of known gender status (Krause, 2021). Such underlying aspects like individual and relational protective factors (e.g., identity resilience, self-efficacy, quality of support from friends, and significant others) that further shape guilt and shame and sense of self-worth, not considered in the present study, could be responsible for negative correlation obtained between shame, guilt, and self-esteem responses obtained during the COVID-19 period. The statistically significant Kendall's TauB correlation value obtained for the association between shame-guilt and self-esteem supported the proposed alternative hypothesis, indicating a significant relationship between these two variables.

With the growing acceptance of the LGBTQIA+ community in India, it becomes essential to acknowledge their concerns related to social inclusion. This study attempted to understand a basic yet curious question of whether shame and guilt are more prominent amongst heterosexual men and women or the LGBTQIA+ community. The present findings indicate that LGBTQIA+ people who have accepted their sexual orientation or gender identity and feel validated in their identity may have similar levels of self-esteem as heterosexual people. Probable factors behind the similarity of LGBTQIA+ and heterosexual groups' self-esteem scores, could be the similarity of support systems for both groups during the COVID-19 period (Gonzales et al., 2023).

Limitations

While the current study findings affirmed the existing research evidence about the overall relationship between shame, guilt, and self-esteem amongst sexual minority and heterosexual group members, the findings specifically from this study lack the power of generalisability as the scores of shame and guilt deviate significantly from the norm.

Besides, the lens of examination of all three variables in the study adopted a heteronormative approach, i.e., a universally accepted socio-generic framework instead of a gender-specific one. Gender-specific or gender-driven approaches to understanding shame, guilt, and self-esteem would perhaps generate a clearer picture of the interplay between the variables. As already outlined earlier, existing research literature proved that the interplay between these variables is rather a seemingly multicomplex phenomenon and certainly involves the role of other mediating or moderating protective factors (both individual and relational) which were not kept in the purview of this study.

Implications and Suggestions

It is recommended that future studies also consider taking a gender-oriented approach for shame, guilt, and self-esteem constructs instead of a heteronormative one to get a detailed understanding of how affiliation with a certain gender identity impacts one's self-conscious emotions. Gender-oriented tools for measuring shame and guilt are also therefore a requirement in this direction.

Since prevailing literature distinguished shame and guilt with the latter as having a more negative impact on self-esteem, studies in future could consider both constructs as two distinct variables of influence.

Community groups or societies or representatives of LGBTQIA+ individuals can take note of the findings and emphasise more on active and supportive community group cohesion and promote social awareness campaigns challenging the stereotypes against the communities while encouraging acceptance towards the sexual minority in the country. Similarly, in the education setting, the modules or the programmes should cater for the sensitivity towards the LGBTQIA+ community which will be a strong support system holistically. Social support campaigns and drives especially in crisis events of pandemics, famine, drought, war, etc. would certainly ensure the wellbeing of the marginalised minority group members who otherwise face challenges in vocalising their needs and concerns.

Conclusion

The current study aimed to study the differences between heterosexual men and women and the LGBTQIA+ community in the context of shame, guilt, and self-esteem. A total of 130 individuals participated. The Guilt Shame Questionnaire was used to measure Shame and Guilt levels, and RSES scale was used to measure the self-esteem of individuals. There were found to be no significant differences in shame, guilt, and self-esteem amongst heterosexual men and women and the LGBTQIA+ group members thereby, rejecting the first two alternate hypotheses of the study. The shame and guilt would share an inverse relationship for all participants irrespective of their gender status. In a nutshell, the present study was able to conclude that shame and guilt experiences during the COVID-19 pandemic had an adverse impact on the self-esteem of members from LGBTQIA+ and heterosexual group members.

References

Anderson, J. R., & Koc, Y. (2020). Identity integration as a protective factor against guilt and shame for religious gay men. *The Journal of Sex Research, 57*(8), 1059–1068. https://doi.org/10.1080/00224499.2020.1767026

Banerjee, D., & Nair, V. S. (2020). "The untold side of COVID-19": Struggle and perspectives of the sexual minorities. *Journal of Psychosexual Health, 2*(2), 113–120. https://doi.org/10.1177/2631831820939017

Breakwell, D. G. (2020). In the age of societal uncertainty, the era of threat. *Frontiers in Sociology and Social Research* (pp. 55–71). Springer. https://doi.org/10.1007/978-3-030-39315-1_6

Breakwell, G. M., & Jaspal, R. (2022). Coming out, distress and identity threat in gay men in the UK. *Sexuality Research and Social Policy*, *19*(3), 1166–1177. https://doi.org/10.1007/s13178-021-00608-4

Budiarto, Y., & Helmi, A. F. (2021). Shame and self-esteem: a meta-analysis. *Europe's Journal of Psychology*, *17*(2), 131–145. https://doi.org/10.5964/ejop.2115

Cabral, J., & Pinto, T. M. (2023). Gender, shame, and social support in LGBTQI+ exposed to discrimination: A model for understanding the impact on mental health. *Social Sciences*, *12*(8), 454. https://doi.org/10.3390/socsci12080454

Choi, H. (2024). Integrating guilt and shame into the self-concept: The influence of future opportunities. *Behavioral Sciences*, *14*(6), 472. https://doi.org/10.3390/bs14060472

Das, H. K., & Govindappa, L. (2023). Anxiety, depression and social support of LGBTQI during COVID-19 in Kerala, India. *International Journal of Social Psychiatry*, *69*(8), 1971–1978. https://doi.org/10.1177/00207640231183913

Datta, S., & Mukherjee, T. (2023). Impact of COVID-19 stress on the psychological health of sexual & gender minority individuals: A systematic review. *Frontiers in Global Women's Health*, *4*, 1132768.https://doi.org/10.3389/fgwh.2023.1132768

Devi, S. (1977). *The World of Homosexuals*. Vikas Publishing House.

Dyvik, E. (2024, October 15). LGBTQ+ worldwide statistics & facts. *Personality & Behavior*. www.statista.com/topics/8579/lgbtq-worldwide/#topicOverview

Gil, R. M., Freeman, T. L., Mathew, T., Kullar, R., Fekete, T., Ovalle, A., Nguyen, D., Kottkamp, A., Poon, J., Marcelin, J. R., & Swartz, T. H. (2021). Lesbian, gay, bisexual, transgender, and Queer (LGBTQ+) Communities and the Coronavirus Disease 2019 pandemic: A call to break the cycle of structural barriers. *The Journal of Infectious Diseases*, *224*(11), 1810–1820. https://doi.org/10.1093/infdis/jiab392

Gonzales, G., de Mola, E. L., Robertson, L., Gavulic, K. A., & McKay, T. (2023). LGBTQ College student health and wellbeing at the onset of the pandemic: Additional evidence and lessons learned from COVID-19. *BMX Public Health*, *23*(1), 967.https://doi.org/10.1186/s12889-023-15909-z

Hoppen, T. H., Schlechter, P., Arntz, A., Rameckers, S. A., Ehring, T., & Morina, N. (2022). A brief measure of guilt and shame: Validation of the Guilt and Shame Questionnaire (GSQ-8). *European Journal of Psychotraumatology*, *13*(2), 1–13. https://doi.org/10.1080/20008066.2022.2146720

IPSOS. (2021). LGBT+ Pride 2021 global survey: A global generation gap around gender identity and sexual attraction. *IPSOS*. www.ipsos.com/sites/default/files/ct/news/documents/2021-06/LGBT%20Pride%202021%20Global%20Survey%20Report_0.pdf

Kidd, J. D., Jackman, K. B., Wolff, M., Veldhuis, C. B., & Hughes, T. L. (2018). Risk and protective factors for substance use among sexual and gender minority youth: A scoping review. *Current Addiction Reports*, *5*(2), 158–173. https://doi.org/10.1007/s40429-018-0196-9

Kline, N. S. (2020). Rethinking COVID-19 vulnerability: A call for LGBTQ+ im/migrant health equity in the United States during and after a pandemic. *Health Equity*, *4*(1), 239–242. https://doi.org/10.1089/heq.2020.0012

Krause, K. D. (2021). Implications of the COVID-19 pandemic on LGBTQI communities. *Journal of Public Health Management and Practice*, *27*(Supplement 1), S69–S71. https://doi.org/10.1097/phh.0000000000001273

Li, H., Liu, X., Zheng, Q., Zeng, S., & Luo, X. (2023). Minority stress, social support and mental health among lesbian, gay, and bisexual college students in China: A moderated mediation analysis. *BMC Psychiatry*, *23*(1), 1–14.https://doi.org/10.1186/s12888-023-05202-z

Luthar, S. S., Crossman, E. J., & Small, P. J. (2015). Resilience and adversity. *Handbook of Child Psychology and Developmental Science: Socioemotional Processes* (7th ed., pp. 247–286). John Wiley & Sons, Inc. https://doi.org/10.1002/9781118963418.childpsy307

Mink, M. D., Lindley, L. L., & Weinstein, A. A. (2014). Stress, stigma, and sexual minority status: The intersectional ecology model of LGBTQ health. *Journal of Gay & Lesbian Social Services*, *26*(4), 502–521. https://doi.org/10.1080/10538720.2014.953660

Mishra, J. (2020). Queering emotion in South Asia: Biographical narratives of gay men in Odisha, India. *Asian Journal of Social Science*, *48*(3/4), 353–374. www.jstor.org/stable/27076295

Mohan, K. (2022). Indian LGBTQ+ youth: The 'invisible' orientations and mental health. *International Journal of Indian Psychology*, *10*(2), 429–44523. https://doi.org/10.25215/1002.044

Monteiro, R. P., De Holanda Coelho, G. L., Hanel, P. H. P., De Medeiros, E. D., & Da Silva, P. D. G. (2021). The efficient assessment of self-esteem: Proposing the brief Rosenberg Self-Esteem Scale. *Applied Research in Quality of Life*, *17*(2), 931–947. https://doi.org/10.1007/s11482-021-09936-4

Ovesen, N. (2023). Layers of shame: The impact of shame in lesbian and Queer Victim-Survivors' accounts of violence and help-seeking. *Journal of Family Violence, 39*, 1365–1377. https://doi.org/10.1007/s10896-023-00626-3

Pachankis, J. E., Hatzenbuehler, M. L., Klein, D. N., & Bränström, R. (2024). The role of shame in the sexual-orientation disparity in mental health: A prospective population-based study of multimodal emotional reactions to stigma. *Clinical Psychological Science*, *12*(3), 486–504. https://doi.org/10.1177/21677026231177714

Peters, J. R., Mereish, E. H., Krek, M. A., Chuong, A., Ranney, M. L., Solomon, J., Spirito, A., & Yen, S. (2019). Sexual orientation differences in non-suicidal self-injury, suicidality, and psychosocial factors among an inpatient psychiatric sample of adolescents. *Psychiatry Research, 284*, 112664. https://doi.org/10.1016/j.psychres.2019.112664

Rapinda, K. K., Pchajek, J., Edgerton, J. D., & Keough, M. T. (2021). Coping with shame mediates the association between depression and gambling severity and frequency. *International Journal of Mental Health and Addiction*, *20*(3), 1645–1658. https://doi.org/10.1007/s11469-020-00469-9

Rosenberg, M. (1965). *Society and the Adolescent Self-Image*. Princeton University Press.

Scheer, J. R., Harney, P., Esposito, J., & Woulfe, J. M. (2020). Self-reported mental and physical health symptoms and potentially traumatic events among lesbian, gay, bisexual, transgender, and queer individuals: The role of shame. *Psychology of Violence*, *10*(2), 131–142. https://doi.org/10.1037/vio0000241

Stotzer, R. L., Ka'opua, L. S., & Diaz, T. P. (2014). Is healthcare caring in Hawai'i? Preliminary results from a health assessment of lesbian, gay, bisexual, transgender, questioning, and intersex people in four counties. *Hawai'i Journal of Medicine & Public Health: A Journal of Asia Pacific Medicine & Public Health*, *73*(6), 175–180. Pubmed. https://pubmed.ncbi.nlm.nih.gov/24959391/

10 Executive Summary

From Editor's Pen [Keyboard]

Rajesh Verma

Introduction

Before introducing the book, let me begin with a rich excerpt from the spiritual classic 'Autobiography of a Yogi' about one of the women saints of India who stopped eating at the tender age of 12 years and 4 months until she left her mortal body (Yogananda, 1975). Below is the reply to a question about her life by the sage-cum-writer Sh. Paramahansa Yogananda to Giri Bala, the woman saint. Below is the response of Giri Bala, the woman saint to Sh. Paramahansa Yogananda who posed a question regarding her life.

> I was born in these forest regions. My childhood was unremarkable save that I was possessed by an insatiable appetite. I had been betrothed in early years. Child, my mother often warned me, try to control your greed. When the time comes for you to live among strangers in your husband's family, what will they think of you if your days are spent in nothing but eating? The calamity she had foreseen came to pass. I was only twelve when I joined my husband's people in Nawabganj. My mother-in-law shamed me morning, noon, and night about my gluttonous habits. Her scoldings were a blessing in disguise, however; they roused my dormant spiritual tendencies. One morning her ridicule was merciless. I shall soon prove to you, I said, stung to the quick, that I shall never touch food again as long as I live. My mother-in-law laughed in derision. So! She said, how can you live without eating, when you cannot live without overeating? This remark was unanswerable! Yet an iron resolution scaffolded my spirit. In a secluded spot I sought my Heavenly Father. Lord, I prayed incessantly, please send me a guru, one who can teach me to live by Thy light and not by food. A divine ecstasy fell over me. Led by a beatific spell, I set out for the Nawabganj ghat on the Ganges. The morning sun pierced the waters; I purified myself in the Ganges, as though for a sacred initiation. As I left the river bank, my wet cloth around me, in the broad glare of day my master materialised himself before me! Dear little one, he said in a voice of loving compassion, I am the guru sent here by God to fulfil your urgent prayer. From today you shall live by the astral light, your bodily atoms fed from the infinite current. He initiated me into a kria technique which frees the body from dependence on the gross food of mortals. The

DOI: 10.4324/9781003517313-11

technique includes the use of a certain mantra and a breathing exercise more difficult than the average person could perform. No medicine or magic is involved; nothing beyond the kria.

(Yogananda, 1975, pp. 502–504)

It is interesting to note here that how Giri Bala who was fond of eating could override the calamity she faced at in-laws house. Though she managed it in an unusual way, but she managed in her own typical style. The calamities not only cause challengeable difficulties but also awaken the dormant energies. She was hurt not physically but psychologically which was so deep that it forced her to take the 'Bhishma Pratijya'[1]which she kept till the end. An intense need to overcome the gluttonous habit aroused in her. The physiological craving turned into psychological pandemic which made her to respond to it in her unique style. She faced her psychological crisis alone and triumphed while the world collectively battled the COVID-19 pandemic and attempting to come out of it even almost half a decade after. As Giri Bala's eating habit acted as blessing in disguise similarly COVID-19 pandemic was blessing in disguise where it accelerated the healthcare sector (Vahia & Shah, 2020) and opened a fresh 'window of options to deal with the environmental degradation' (Verma, 2022, p. 216).

The book has compiled studies that attempted to demystify the profound psychological impact of COVID-19 pandemic on the specific population of India and ensuing needs. The specific population means studies done on particular segment of society such as, women survivors, married women, youth, adults, children, elderly, asexuals, students, and female domestic workers. The pandemic helped in creating an informed awareness about importance of mental health (Verma, 2024) in the erstwhile India where it was the last item on the healthcare list. The idea of focussing on the specific Indian population was to highlight the impact and varying coping mechanisms used in context of cultural diversity of India.

No doubt all suffered but at varying degree attributed to the strength of mental health. For example, Gaur et al. (2021) found that urban area students experienced heightened fear of COVID-19 infection than their rural counterparts. The women faced heightened domestic violence at the initial phase of pandemic (Maji et al., 2022) and excessive domestic workload. The elderly had their own challenges such as 'perceived apprehension of adverse course of existing morbidity' (Vahia & Shah, 2020, p. 1) neglect, insecurity, and fear (Khatri et al., 2023) extreme fatigue (Diyali, 2023). The children and adolescent faced screen dependency, drop-outs, worsening gender gaps in education (Kumar et al., 2020), online shaming, and self-promotion through social media (Behra et al., 2022).It was pandemic that made the youth to rediscover and revitalise the significance of interpersonal relations, social connections, and support. The challenges of COVID-19 led to self-suspiciousness and heightened vigilance regarding personal hygiene. Certainly, the challenges of COVID-19 were typical, unique, and harsh, yet they also opened doors to new learning, coping strategies, ways of living, studying, meeting, interacting, and cognitive–behavioural reappraisal (Verma, 2022). Some of the major needs of Indians that can be uniquely attributed to post-COVID-19 milieu include close affiliation, pro-active health management measures, importance of home cooked food, happiness one of the most preferred component of one's day-to-day behaviour and appreciation of universal human values. In this backdrop, it was essential to assess, investigate, and compile the mental, emotional, and behavioural health needs of the specific population of India in one volume which contains nine chapters. Below is a summary of each chapter:

Executive Summary

Chapter 1: "At What Point Should I Bring Up My Asexuality?" Lived Experiences of *Asexuals in the Post-Pandemic Era*

The Million Killer and Billions Scarer (COVID-19) marched like a dust storm through the convoy human beings and carried with it whoever came in the way. It showed its presence either by inflicting or by instilling the fear of infection. The intensity of fear can be gauged from the fact that some of the researchers named it as 'coronaphobia' (Arora et al., 2020; Asmundson & Taylor, 2020; Lee & Crunk, 2022). The 'fear tsunami' also gripped the asexuals one of the excommunicated minority societies. They faced the double whammy where they had some socially acceptance-related issues while COVID-19 compounded their already burdened cognitive system. The asexuals narrated how they felt to be isolated and irrelevant during and after the COVID-19 waves. The feelings of social rejection when everyone was searching for social support is likely to be detrimental for mental health and asexuals faced this bizarre situation. This particular study found that the asexuals devised mechanism to deal with the distressing situations by coming up with two situation handling strategies such as 'drawing boundaries' and seeking professional help. Drawing boundaries means limiting expressions, reactions, responses, and interactions. Their unique necessity compelled them to devise 'self'-specific means to handle adverse situations and maintaining and managing their mental health. The second strategy was to seek professional help. While not new but it is the best course when in rough weather. In close social circuits, as practiced in several cultures, seeking professional help is no less than a courageous effort. India being cultural hub that had a spectrum of societies ranging from tightly knit communities to more open Western type societies provides a unique backdrop. From the participants' narratives, two important points worth attention emerged. The excessive lack of awareness in society about asexuals and undeclared social compulsion of marriage. In light of these themes, the authors discussed the idea of the need for the development of a positive self-concept by asexuals and the major potential social challenges of recognition of asexuals as one of the components of society. Before recognition, society should accept the fact that such people do exist within the ambit of social structure. The natural outcome of recognition will be acceptance and ensuing changes. The chapter concludes by asserting that academia and society can be instrumental in initiating a discussion to accommodate and accept asexuals as a mandatory colour of society's rainbow.

Chapter 2: Psychological Impact of Institutional Quarantine on Border Security Force Personnel of India

The typical English word 'quarantine', with its characteristic tongue-and-lip rolling pronunciation, evolved from medieval port cities, where it was reserved for ships coming from bubonic plague-hit ports. Pre-COVID-19, it was a key and commonly use term in public health lexicon. However, post-COVID-19, it became the dread word for common people across the globe. Interestingly, the unprecedented spread of COVID-19 brought the age-old strategy of quarantine to the forefront, proving essential in containing the spread and proving instrumental in directing modern global health policies. The chapter, 'Psychological Impact of Institutional Quarantine on Border Security Force Personnel' had attempted to decipher the impact on psycho-physically hardened force of India. The evidence suggests that people who were quarantined during the pandemic were at the heightened risk of developing anxiety and depression. The studies observed that post-traumatic stress symptoms, confusion, and anger were most commonly seen mental health issues among people who were forced to remain quarantined. The role of Border Security Forces is very complex that involves assembly and continuous close physical coordination among a group of soldiers. The assembly of individuals is easy fodder for the COVID-19. Hence, the border security faced a complex challenge in balancing dual responsibilities: maintaining high levels of security while simultaneously combating COVID-19. To address this, institutional quarantine centres were established to isolate infected personnel. However, this approaches had unintended consequences, notably exacerbating psychological problems among quarantined soldiers, which underscores the critical impact of quarantine on mental health within high-stress environments. The study used cross-sectional observational design to assess the impact on 176 Border Security Force personnel of both genders using standardised tools such as Impact of Event Scale, Beck Depression Inventory-II, State Trait Anxiety Inventory, and Perceived Stress Scale along with interview schedule. The findings indicated that the level of subjective distress, depression was relatively very low. The participants experienced moderate to high level of anxiety with lower level of stress. The correlation analysis suggests that the subjective distress had significant positive association with depression, anxiety, and perceived stress. The findings suggest that depression and anxiety have positive correlation and similar is the case with anxiety and stress. The regression outcomes indicate those individuals who perceive stress and suffer from subjective distress are likely to develop depression and anxiety. In conclusion, the typicality associated with the life style of Border Security Force personnel acted as psychological shield which is vindicated by the findings of this study. The authors attribute the results to the role of institutional training in mitigating the negative impact of institutional quarantine.

Chapter 3: Impact of COVID-19 and Social Distancing Measures on Married Women: A Qualitative Enquiry

While going through this chapter, I was reminded of Khalil Gibran's words in his classic, 'The Prophet' about marriage where he says, 'Fill each other's cup but drink not from one cup. And stand together yet not too near together'. Married women, one of the most important pillars of social structure, have their own challenges, responsibilities, and conveniences. This chapter has delved to understand how the mobility restrictions affected those women who are married and staying with their in-laws during the pandemic times. Not even the governments who imposed the mobility restrictions to contain the spread thought that it may have adverse effect on the lives of married women. They faced several challenges including unending domestic responsibilities, care-burden, lost-individuality, domestic violence, financial dependency, disruption of routine, almost no physical social-life, sedentary and dull life, enhanced psycho-physical labour, feeling of being immured, gadget operating dependency, and others. The added psychosocial burden tends to compromise the mental health which married women faced during the infamous lockdowns. The telephonic interviews of married women (22–45 years) yielded interesting insights which were analysed by thematic analysis. The few of the themes that emerged includes 'emotional and psychological impact', 'social impact', 'impact on workload', and 'coping'. These themes are more deeply explained with supporting verbatim narrations. Each theme has been explained through the finer contents such as anxiety, gender inequalities, conflicts, and dilemmas. The prolonged lockdowns, lasting nearly six months during both waves, compelled women to adapt to new challenges. They employed various coping mechanisms customised to their unique psychosocial circumstances. Habituation and forced adjustment were few that emerged from the narratives of the small sample. On the other hand, the lockdowns did not have all negative impacts,it has positive ones too where few of the respondents shared that it was a good time to know my husband from close quarters, else he was busy with his work and had less time for family. Some were lucky to get support in household chores from their husbands. The authors carefully curetted the transcriptions for their contents and presented in a systematic style.

Chapter 4: Resilience Amidst Adversity: Exploration of Undergraduate Students Post-COVID-19 Experiences in Kerala

'Student' is a nostalgic word which reminds me of different levels of teens dressed in the latest trend with two or three books thrust into the lap of their left hand, sipping some hot stuff while engaging in loud laughter even on non-laughable events. The enigmatic COVID-19 pandemic left every segment of society perplexed and people had so much of mixed yet unique experiences which need approximately a million of pages to record. In this backdrop, this study explored the undergraduate students' experiences keeping the 'resilience' as focal point. From the standpoint of psychology,'resilience' is a one of the survival construct-cum-ability of human beings. The level of resilience has direct impact upon the mental health. The study was conducted on 85 students from different graduate streams representing 50% districts (7) of Kerala. The study was designed to understand the role of resilience in coping with the COVID-19 led challenges and to explore the different coping mechanisms used by this particular class of society. The study reported that more than half of students revealed high level of resilience, one-fifth reported average and one-fourth reported low level. The resilience was assessed using Mowbray (2014) Resilience Assessment Questionnaire (RAQ). The findings point out that students who maintained social connectedness, had positive psychological traits found to have high resilience. And, higher the resilience betters the mental health (Sood & Sharma, 2020). Sharing among peers, social support, online discussions, mutual collaborations, and reciprocated emotional support played significant role in handling the adversity effectively. Interestingly, the virtual support also played significant role in coping and strengthening the resilience. One of the important qualities that helped the students in mitigating the adverse impact of COVID-19 on mental health was cognitive flexibility of the students. Curiosity is one of the traits of students which allows them to seek all kinds of help in need, also helped them in keeping their feet firm. Concluding the findings authors suggests that effective interaction and organisation are indispensable tools for navigating challenges.

Chapter 5: Psychological After-Effects of COVID-19 among Women Survivors of *Maharashtra, India*

Bwire (2020, p. 874) cited that 'The epidemiological findings reported across different parts of the world indicated higher morbidity and mortality in males than females'. Women tends to bear the highest brunt of calamities (Bhadra, 2024) and have higher mortality, i.e., 14 times more than men (Okai, 2022). Interestingly, during the COVID-19 pandemic among those infected with the virus, the women excelled in survival rate over men (Gerdeman, 2020). Various factors might contribute to this gender disparity, though only a few disparities tend to favour women. The study focused on this section of population who fighting with all sorts of odd and proved their psycho-physiological mettle. 304 women from the second largest city of Maharashtra participated and telephonically interviewed using the PTSD checklist which contained 21 items. The PTSD checklist was administered during a period ranging from 1 month to 12 months after recovery. The study revealed two major symptoms 'being super alert about COVID-19' and 'avoiding external reminders of COVID-19 illness'. The symptoms were indicative of mental health status. The prevalence of PTSD among the sample was much lower than the global trend. However, the distribution of distress varied in women based on socio-economic status, employment status, and treatment centres status (isolation wards, quarantine centres, or home) during the pandemic. The low prevalence of distress is probably due to the socio-cultural factors such as collectivism, close interpersonal associations, joint family system, spread all around and stronger relational bonding, virtual sharing of hardships, and freely venting out feelings to friends and families and emotive social support, all of which likely strengthened the resilience which probably shielded the mental health of participating women. The concluding remarks suggests that socio-demographic factors were significant contributors in manifestation of distress symptoms and those who spent time in quarantine centres took longer time for recovery and faced higher level of distress.

Chapter 6: Browsing to Worrying in Post-COVID Era: Quantifying the Links between Internet Addiction, Cyberchondria, and Health Anxiety in Emerging Adults of North-East India

The internet, specifically post-COVID-19 pandemic, has fundamentally altered the paradigms of human interaction and several aspects of human behaviour. In terms of mental health, internet has added a new psychological concern to an already overflowing basket of mental health issues. This concern is technically known as cyberchondria which refers to compulsive and problematic internet search for health-related information such as symptoms, diagnoses, and treatments. The cyberchondria is an offshoot of excessive use and consequent reliance on the internet, which is closely related to internet addiction. This chapter explores the correlations among cyberchondria, internet addiction, and health anxiety among most vulnerable population to problematic internet use, i.e., emerging adults belonging to North-East India. The combined and independently all three variables are a potent threat to the psychological wellbeing of problematic internet users. 371 emerging adults (18–25 years) were selected from the Arunachal Pradesh, Assam, Meghalaya, Mizoram, Manipur, Nagaland, Tripura, and Sikkim and assessed for the three variables using Cyberchondria Severity Scale, Internet Addiction Test, and Health Anxiety Inventory. The data were collected through online mode. The findings showed that cyberchondria, internet addiction, and health have a kind of give and take relationship which means that cyberchondriacs are likely to fall in the trap of internet addiction and excessive health-related searches. The findings also reveal the cyclical connection between the selected variables where excessive health-related browsing leads to increased anxiety, which in turn leads to problematic internet use thereby creating a feedback loop from which it is not easy to escape. The results further showed that marital status also have a significant role in cyberchondriasis and higher level of health-related anxiety. One of the major limitations of the study is that it has limited to specific population, i.e., emerging adults of North-East India. The authors concluded by stressing upon the need for development of potent interventions that can address the problematic internet use to promote healthy online functioning to circumvent the getting trapped into the vicious cycle of internet addiction and health related anxiety.

Chapter 7: Unveiling the Experiences of Women Domestic Workers in India amid and beyond the COVID-19 Pandemic: A Narrative Review

Domestic workers is a one of the specific social groups that employs more than 5 crore (50 million) people in India. Due to several factors such as legal instruments, social protection, job security, labour issues, other employment benefits, and others, these workers are in the informal sector which makes them vulnerable to various kinds of psycho-physical and social exploitation. In India, it is estimated that almost two-third of domestic workers are employed in urban areas (Sumalatha et al., 2021) and women make it 80% of this workforce (Domestic Workers Rights

Movement, n. d.). Most of the women domestic workers who are either full-time or part-time prefer daily up and down from their makeshift homes to their workplace. The mobility restrictions during the COVID-19 adversely affected their job perspectives and consequently their incomes. Considering the comprehensive impact of the COVID-19 pandemic on this vulnerable group this study through narrative analysis reviewed the studies that were conducted on the topic and published from March 2020 to April 2024. The authors searched all major electronic databases for the targeted literature. Finally, zeroed it down to eight studies that altogether amount to a total sample of 1111 women domestic workers, which are systematically placed in the table. The included studies covered 13 different cities spanning across India. The major findings of the reviewed literature includes job loss, financial hardship, marital stress, insecurity at multiple levels, post-pandemic stigmatisation, gendered domestic violence and discrimination, insomniac symptoms, trust deficit, healthcare issues, reproductive health issues, decline in nutrient intake, increased debt, post-pandemic increased domestic workload, increased stress and health problems, and care burden. Apart from negative impact, there was a ray of hope shared by the sample. To some extent, employer and government support helped in mitigating their wows. The findings are discussed in a hierarchical setup starting with pre-existing vulnerabilities to impact of the pandemic on employment and income, health, occupational risks, and safety concerns, social stigma and isolation, domestic stress, and care burden amidst the pandemic, and navigating the post-pandemic terrain: challenges so far. The author concluded by highlighting the plight of women domestic workers during the pandemic and post-pandemic which needs to be first acknowledged at the highest level which might pave the way for addressing their psycho-social and of course financial concerns.

Chapter 8: Neuro-Divergence and COVID-19 Pandemic: A Reflexive Thematic Analysis on the Experiences of a Mother of An Autistic Child

The term 'neurodivergence' connotes the presence of some typical brain-related condition that needs specialised attention. Autism is a condition which is identified with intellectual limitations and social-communication inhibition. ICD-11 states that 'Individuals with Autism Spectrum Disorder may exhibit limitations in intellectual abilities' (ICD-11 for Mortality and Morbidity Statistics, n.d.). The chapter starts with a positive note for the people who suffer from autism, which is one of the neurodivergent types where it mentions that autism is not a deficiency but rather a human rights issue. The chapter contextualised autism as a challenge and proceeded to thematically analyse the experiences gained through the telephonic interview of a 43-year-old mother, who is the caregiver, of an autistic child. The authors typically start with a historical examination of parents' health, and pre- and post-natal conditions and share the vital demographics, essential for establishing the credibility of the study. The mother had a normal pregnancy; the child had normal motor development but faced some difficulties in social development. The psychometric assessment of the child provided evidence of the 'dull average' category and subsequently, the child displayed mild Autism Spectrum Disorders symptoms. Though, it was not a piece of good news for parents, their total acceptance of the child proved instrumental in managing the uncalled-for situation. The management of child during the normal times (Pre-COVID-19) was relatively easier but the unfortunate mobility restrictions shifted the care burden to the mother which proved to be challenging and testing. Data were collected using a 10-item open-ended questionnaire. The analysis of responses revealed five major themes: resilience in adversity, struggles with social isolation, adaptation and creativity, advocacy for change, and hope and resilience for the future. The themes are discussed within the context of existing literature. The findings conclude that COVID-19 shifted the care burden and increased the diversity of challenges for the mother of the neurodivergent child. However, parents employed ingenious methods and coping strategies to manage the unprecedented situation created by the COVID-19 pandemic.

Chapter 9: Pandemic and Pride: Shame, Guilt, and Self-Esteem in LGBTQIA+ and Heterosexual Individuals

The diversity of sexual orientation is one of the unique characteristics of humans. The existence of LGBTQIA+ people are representative of sexual orientation diversity. This community has rich history of struggle to be recognised as part of mainstream life. Despite their efforts and legal security, they still feel stigmatised, isolated, adjustment issues, complex trauma, frequent feeling of guilt and shame by virtue of being under the umbrella of LGBTQIA+ term. Evidence suggests that the acceptance rate of these people is being improved. Under these challenging circumstances and additional challenges posed by the COVID-19 pandemic, this community faced some peculiar situations which are being attempted to address in the present study which is explored the psychological impacts of the COVID-19 pandemic on diversified sexual orientation. 130 participants (17–42 years) equally divided between heterosexual and self-identified LGBTQIA+ group included various identities, predominantly bisexual, gay, and lesbian selected through online platforms supplemented by snowball and peer referencing techniques. The central theme was to assess the levels of shame, guilt, and self-esteem among both categories of people. The findings revealed no significant differences in shame, guilt, and self-esteem between the LGBTQIA+ community and heterosexual individuals. The results are encouraging and relief giving which says that both groups experienced similar levels of these emotions during the pandemic for social outcast minority considering the outcomes. Further, an inverse correlation was seen between shame, guilt, and self-esteem, which indicate that higher levels of shame and guilt were associated with lower self-esteem. One of the major limitations was that sampling was purposive and self-identified orientation. Authors concluded by highlighting the psychological challenges faced by both LGBTQIA+ and heterosexual individuals during the COVID-19 pandemic, showing that the experiences of shame and guilt are prevalent across different sexual orientations.

Conclusion

And, the current trend and direction of growth of science and technology is the indicative to human race of many more COVID-19 like pandemics in near future. So, writings, findings, and discussion may be of some help, but we need to be future ready to be psychologically strong and mentally tough to face the impending dangers. Here, I may seem to be pessimistic, yet it is nothing less than our face in mirror.

Acknowledgements

I sincerely thank all my contributors on whose work this chapter has been built up, without their contributions it was not possible to come up with this chapter. It would be unfair on my part if I fail to express my gratitude to my wife Dr Sujit Verma for giving me ideas and helping me in structuring this work.

Note

1 In the great epic Mahabharata, Bhishma, the revered great-grandfather of Pandavas and Kauravas, took a vow to remain unmarried and celibate for his entire life. This harsh and tough vow is popularly known as Bhishma Pratijya.

References

American Psychiatric Association. (2013). *Diagnostic and Statistical Manual of Mental Disorders,* 5th Ed. Washington, DC: American Psychiatric Publishing.

Arora, A., Jha, A. K., Alat, P., & Das, S. S. (2020). Understanding coronaphobia . *Asian Journal of Psychiatry, 54*, 102384. https://doi.org/10.1016/j.ajp.2020.102384

Asmundson, G. J. G., & Taylor, S. (2020). Coronaphobia revisited: A state-of-the-art on pandemic-related fear, anxiety, and stress. *Journal of Anxiety Disorders, 76*, 102326. https://doi.org/10.1016/j.janxdis.2020.102326

Behera, R. K., Bala, P. K., Rana, N. P., & Kayal, G. (2022). Self-promotion and online shaming during COVID-19: A toxic combination. *International Journal of Information Management Data Insights*, *2*(2), 100117. https://doi.org/10.1016/j.jjimei.2022.100117

Bhadra, R. (2024, June 17). *Unveiling the Disproportionate Impact: Women in the Shadow of Disasters.* Her Zindagi. www.msn.com/en-in/news/India /unveiling-the-disproportionate-impact-women-in-the-shadow-of-disasters/ar-BB1onjKi?ocid=msedgntp&pc=U531&cvid=5ccd3a709d644590979d927f87c42066&ei=13

Bwire, G. M. (2020). Coronavirus: Why men are more vulnerable to Covid-19 than women?. *SN Comprehensive Clinical Medicine*, *2*(7), 874–876. https://doi.org/10.1007/s42399-020-00341-w

Diyali, C. (2023). Second wave of corona and elderly mental health in India: Challenges and way forward. In: M.K. Shankardass (Eds), *Handbook on COVID-19 Pandemic and Older Persons*. Springer, Singapore. https://doi.org/10.1007/978-981-99-1467-8_40

Domestic Workers Movement in India (n.d.). Global Fund for Women. Retrieved June 26, 2024, from www.globalfundforwomen.org/movements/domestic-workers-rights-movement/

Gaur, G., Sharma, M., Kundu, M., Sekhon, H., & Chauhan, N. (2021). Fear of COVID-19 among the Indian youth: A cross-sectional study. *Journal of Education and Health Promotion, 10,* 340. https://doi.org/10.4103/jehp.jehp_1455_20

Gerdeman, D. (2020, October 20). *The COVID Gender Gap: Why Fewer Women Are Dying [Review of The COVID Gender Gap: Why Fewer Women Are Dying].* Business Research for Business Leaders. https://hbswk.hbs.edu/item/the-covid-gender-gap-why-fewer-women-are-dying

Gross, J. J., & John, O. P. (2003). Individual differences in two emotion regulation processes: Implications for affect, relationships, and well-being. *Journal of Personality and Social Psychology, 85*(2), 348–362.

Hawkley, L. C., & Cacioppo, J. T. (2010). Loneliness matters: A theoretical and empirical review of consequences and mechanisms. *Annals of Behavioural Medicine: A Publication of the Society of Behavioural Medicine, 40*(2), 218–227. https://doi.org/10.1007/s12160-010-9210-8

Huh, H. J., Kim, K. H., Lee, H. K., Jeong, B. R., Hwang, J. H., & Chae, J. H. (2021). Perceived stress, positive resources and their interactions as possible related factors for depressive symptoms. *Psychiatry Investigation, 18*(1), 59–68. https://doi.org/10.30773/pi.2020.0208

ICD-11 for Mortality and Morbidity Statistics. (n.d.). https://icd.who.int/browse/2024-01/mms/en#437815624

Khatri, K., Vora, P., & De Sousa, A. (2023). COVID-19 and elder abuse: Critical Issues for India. In: M.K. Shankardass (Eds), *Handbook on COVID-19 Pandemic and Older Persons*. Springer, Singapore. https://doi.org/10.1007/978-981-99-1467-8_34

Kumar, M. M., Karpaga, P. P., Panigrahi, S. K., Raj, U., & Pathak, V. K. (2020). Impact of COVID-19 pandemic on adolescent health in India. *Journal of Family Medicine and Primary Care, 9*(11), 5484–5489. https://doi.org/10.4103/jfmpc.jfmpc_1266_20

Lee, S. A., & Crunk, E. A. (2022). Fear and psychopathology during the COVID-19 crisis: Neuroticism, hypochondriasis, reassurance-seeking, and coronaphobia as fear factors. *OMEGA–Journal of Death and Dying, 85*(2), 483–496. https://doi.org/10.1177/0030222820949350

Maji, S., Bansod, S., & Singh, T. (2022). Domestic violence during COVID-19 pandemic: The case for Indian women. *Journal of Community & Applied Social Psychology,* 32(3), 374–381. https://doi.org/10.1002/casp.2501

Mowbray, D. (2014). Strengthening personal resilience. *Management Advisory Service, 24,* 24.

Neff, K. (2003). Self-compassion: An alternative conceptualization of a healthy attitude toward oneself. *Self and Identity, 2*(2), 85–101. https://doi.org/10.1080/1529886030903

Okai, A. (2022, March 24).*Women Are Hit Hardest in Disasters, So Why Are Responses Too Often Gender-Blind?* Retrieved June 18, 2024, from www.undp.org/blog/women-are-hit-hardest-disasters-so-why-are-responses-too-often-gender-blind

Sheldon, C., Tom, K., & Robin, M. (1983). A global measure of perceived stress. *Journal of Health and Social Behavior, 24*(4), 385–396. https://doi.org/10.2307/2136404

Sood, S., & Sharma, A. (2020). Resilience and psychological well-being of higher education students during COVID-19: The mediating role of perceived distress. *Journal of Health Management. 22*(4):606–617. https://doi.org/10.1177/0972063420983111

Sumalatha, B. S., Bhat, L. D., & Chitra, K. P. (2021). Impact of Covid-19 on informal sector: A study of women domestic workers in India . *The Indian Economic Journal, 69*(3), 441–461. https://doi.org/10.1177/00194662211023845

Vahia, V. N., & Shah, A. B. (2020). COVID-19 pandemic and mental health care of older adults in India. *International Psychogeriatrics*, *32*(10), 1125–1127. https://doi.org/10.1017/S1041610220001441

Verma, R. (2022). Responding to COVID-19: A case of psychological response centers. In R. K. Kovid, V. Kumar (Eds), *Cases on Emerging Market Responses to the COVID-19 Pandemic* (pp. 216–241). IGI Global: Hershey. https://doi.org/10.4018/978-1-6684-3504-5.ch011

Verma, R. (2024). Coronavirus: The dreaded avatar that surprised humanity. In R.Verma, U. Uzaina, L. S. S. Manickam, T. Singh, & G. Tiwari (Eds), *Exploring the Psycho-Social Impact of COVID-19: Global Perspectives on Behaviour, Interventions and Future Directions*(pp. 1–18). Routledge: New York.www.routledge.com/Exploring-the-Psycho-Social-Impact-of-COVID-19-Global-Perspectives-on-Behaviour/Verma-Uzaina-Manickam-Singh-Tiwari/p/book/9781003357209

Yogananda, P. (1975). *Autobiography of a Yogi*. Bombay: Jaico.

Index

For Product Safety Concerns and Information please contact our EU representative GPSR@taylorandfrancis.com Taylor & Francis Verlag GmbH, Kaufingerstraße 24, 80331 München, Germany

Batch number: 10397794

Printed by Printforce, the Netherlands